Meal Prep for Beginners:

The Fastest and Most Convenient Cookbook with 50+ Recipes you can get Your Hands on to Prepare Your Meals in a Week Advance to Save Time and Energy! Ready to Go Meals!

Introduction

Congratulations on downloading this book, Meal Prep for Beginners: The Fastest and Most Convenient Cookbook with 50+ Recipes you can get Your Hands on to Prepare Your Meals in a Week Advance to Save Time and Energy! Ready to Go Meals!

Meal prepping can be an overwhelming concept, especially if you are just starting out on your fitness journey. I am here to tell you that you are not alone! First off, let me start by congratulating you on making the decision to lead a healthy life. This alone is a very important first step to take. When you decide to put yourself first, the rest of the benefits will follow.

If you are unaware, there are so many incredible benefits to meal prepping. In the chapters to follow, we will be giving you all of the information you need to get started. The very first chapter will bring light to topics such as: what meal prepping is, some helpful examples, and some of my own tips and tricks to make it even easier. As you will soon find out, some of these benefits are for your health, but they also allow you to save and create time to use in more beneficial ways.

In the chapters after the introduction chapter, you will find 50+ delicious recipes. Whether you are looking to prep breakfast or a simple lunch to bring to work with you, this book has got you covered. Within the chapters, you will find seafood recipes, red meat recipes, chicken recipes, and yes, there is even a dessert recipe. I have tried to include a wide selection for it is a common side effect to become bored of the meals prepped at the beginning of the week. By switching it up every once in a while, it will make it easier to stick to your goals and have it be delicious at the same time!

I am so incredibly happy you have decided to start this journey toward a healthier lifestyle. Whether you are looking to lose weight, gain weight, or maintain your current weight, there is a meal prep plan for absolutely everyone. As you will find in the first chapter, it is completely up to you what you feel your meal prep should include. Every individual is different and will have different tastes. I have made it my duty to include a wide array of recipes to match the desires of just about any person. The recipes vary from easy to moderately difficult, so I highly suggest testing out some of our easier recipes as you dip your toes into the meal prepping life.

By the end of this book, I hope you will feel confident in your meal prepping skills. If it doesn't come across easy the first time, I hope you do not give up. If dieting and meal prepping were easy, everyone would do it. You are strong, and you want this change in your life. All it takes is a little bit of time and some dedication. In the first chapter, you will find some weekly plan examples. These are meant to be a guide, not necessarily need to be followed to a T. I do hope you find the answers you are looking for and enjoy the read.

Additionally, the information in the following pages is intended only for informational purposes and should thus be thought of as universal. As befitting its nature, it is presented without assurance regarding its prolonged validity or interim quality. Trademarks that are mentioned are done without written consent and can in no way be considered an endorsement from the trademark holder.

Chapter One: Introduction to Meal Prep

What is Meal Prepping?

You are here, reading these words right now because you want to learn how to meal prep. The question is, what is meal prepping? Why is meal prepping a thing and how can it benefit your life? While it may seem overwhelming at first, meal prepping can be fun, easy, and eventually saves you a ton of time! The act of meal prepping is to prepare your meals ahead of time, so you don't have to waste more time of your week, just cooking and eating your meals. Instead, you get the cooking out of the way and bring more focus to what is truly important, your health.

If you want to look at it this way, meal prepping is the healthier version of those TV dinners some people love to buy. However, as opposed to being filled with sodium and who knows what kind of fillers, you will be able to prep healthier and unprocessed ingredients. If this seems like too much work, meal prepping may not be for you. But, if you truly want to change your lifestyle and become healthier, meal prepping is the way to go. Nobody claims you have to put the pedal to the metal and get all of your meal preps. Start out slow! Perhaps this week you only prep your breakfast. As you become more comfortable, you can try and prep lunch for the week after. The best part is, there is no wrong way to meal prep! This journey will be your own to fit your own goals. Whether you are looking to lose weight, gain weight, or maintain your weight, there is a meal prepping plan for you.

Getting Started on Meal Prepping

If you are just starting out, your very first goal is not to be overwhelmed. I have seen too many times where people allow themselves to become dragged down by little details that at the end of the day, don't really matter! The secret is to not incorporate too many things at once. This whole concept is brand new to you. You don't have to be an expert level on day one. This will come in time.

Before we start to meal prep, you need to ask yourself what your own personal goals are. Often times, people go on what we call, "health-kicks," and they go all in. When this happens, more time than not, they will quit after a week! Being healthy is a lifestyle, not a quick fix. You are doing this because you have decided to put yourself and your health first. This is so important to remember! Your results won't happen all at once, it is about the journey to the destination. Up to this point, what have your health choices looked like? If you are shaking your head and saying, not very good, that is okay too. Today is a new day. Today, you are choosing to better yourself and learn all about the meal prepping life. Next, you will learn some easy ways to get started.

Choosing Your Day

To start off, you will want to choose a day where you will prepare your meals. For many individuals, Sunday is one of the best days to begin your meal prepping. For most, this day is one that is off from work, and you can spend the time focusing on your meals. If you have a family, perhaps you can try to get them involved! Health is a lifestyle that can be taught to all ages and carry a lesson to be brought through life.

For those who are a bit more experienced, perhaps you would like two days to prep your meals. One of the most popular options includes Sunday and Wednesday. By choosing these two days, this allows people to split up their week and change up their meals. As I said in the introduction, one of the downfalls of meal prep is that people become sick of eating the same foods. By choosing a couple of days, this allows you to switch up your meals and keep things new and tasty.

If you are a beginner, as we all are at one point or another, I highly suggest not prepping a meal for the whole week. If you are just starting out, let's try to start with no more than perhaps three meals. In my opinion, breakfast is one of the more easy meals to prep. If you are like me, waking up in the morning and cooking is not on top of my list. There are too many things to get done, often times not allotting time for a nutritious breakfast. By meal prepping, all you'll have to do is grab, heat, and go. Who wouldn't take the time to do that?

A handy tool I use for my own meal prepping guide is a calendar. If you are a visual learner like I am, this is the perfect way to organize your meals. Whether you use a real calendar or the one of your cell phone, you will have to find out what works best for you. The most important point is that you choose a day or two that fit your schedule, where you can spend the time you need to prep your meals.

Pick Out Your Meals

Now that you have chosen your day, it is time to decide on the meals you want to prepare. As I said earlier, you may want to focus on breakfast first. If you feel you are ready for a more difficult task, go ahead and set your focus to a lunch or a dinner. If you have a family you are feeding, perhaps you will want to put your efforts toward healthy dinners for the whole family. If you are single, lunches may be more important to you. The best part of meal prepping is how flexible the system is. Take the time to focus on your goals and achieve them the best that you are able to.

When you are picking out your meals, try to focus on creating a balance. Health wise, there are three specific macronutrients you should be focused on. These nutrients include fats, carbohydrates, and proteins. As you will find in the recipe part of the section later, we have included all of this information to help you even more on your fitness journey.

We all have different goals when it comes to our fitness journey. Your micronutrients will change whether you are planning on gaining weight, losing weight, or maintaining. You can use any online calculator to decide what your balanced diet should look like. Once this is determined, this will help you choose out your meals. As a basic guide, your meals should include a protein, a carbohydrate, and a fruit and/or vegetable. Look back on your elementary school food pyramid, and you should have a pretty good idea of how to balance your plate.

An extra tool that may help you out with your macronutrients would be a kitchen scale. If you are trying to lose weight and are counting calories, this would be highly beneficial for you. Speaking of tools, this will bring me to my next important tip to successful meal prepping, your containers.

Meal Prepping Containers

Another tool that will be vital to the success of your meal prepping will be your meal prep containers. Think of these containers as the foundation of your meal prepping. There are a few different factors you will want to take into consideration such as size, sections, and material. These will change depending on not only your situation but also your access. If you find that you do not have access to the containers you are looking for at the store, perhaps try online!

When choosing out your containers, try to find ones that are BPA free. In case you were unaware, BPA stands for bisphenol A, which is a very unhealthy industrial chemical found in certain plastics. By being BPA free, your containers will be microwavable, another very important factor in your meal prepping success. As a suggestion, I typically stick with clear containers so I have easy access to what is in each container.

Overall, there is a simple list for you to follow when you are selecting your containers.

1. Dishwasher Safe
2. Microwave Safe
3. Reusable
4. BPA Free
5. Freezer Safe

Making Your List

To begin, as I already said, it is important to start small. Before you even get to the grocery store, try to pick out your meals and create your grocery list. You can do this on paper, or there are plenty of neat apps on your phone to create the lists on. Either way, planning is the key to success. Once you make this list, you will be able to hit the grocery store and purchase what you need.

Step one is figuring out how many meals you will need. For example, if you are prepping all of your meals for the week, you will need fifteen meals. Instead of cooking fifteen separate dishes, try to create large batches of certain foods to use in various ways. By doing this, you are keeping meal prep simple, and it will be easier on you. Sometimes when recipes include too many ingredients, this causes people to shy away from eating healthy. In the chapters to follow, you will see that the recipes are fairly simple yet delicious.

Remember before you start meal prepping that you will be choosing a day to meal prep. If your day is Sunday, perhaps you can do your big shopping on Saturday or earlier that morning. The key is to be organized. When making your list, keep your grocery store in mind. You will want to try your best to organize your list by section such as meat, dairy, produce, etc. This way, you will be able to zip in and out of the store with no issues or distractions.

Meal Prep Tips and Tricks

I understand that meal prepping can be overwhelming. There are new elements such as new foods, new tools, and new ways of cooking foods. As I said, this book is here to help you every step of the way.

1. Find the Time
   We find excuses, it is just a part of human nature. We find any excuse we can to not put ourselves first. We tell ourselves, I'll do it later, or I just don't have the time. It is important to make the time to put the focus on our health. At the end of the day, you will really only need two or three hours to meal prep. As I said earlier, choose your day and stick to the plan. This is absolutely something you can do!
2. Overlap Ingredients
   To make meal prepping a bit easier, try to use ingredients that can overlap and be used in multiple meals. This will save you time and money when you are meal prepping. As you write out your grocery list, think of meals that utilize the same proteins or vegetables. You will thank yourself for making it that much easier by planning ahead.
3. Freezer Friendly
   You may or may not know, but some recipes freeze easier than others. If you plan on prepping your meals for the whole week as opposed to every couple of days, try to cook meals you can pop in the freezer. Some examples of this would be brothers, soups, and smoothies. These are especially good when you are short on time and find yourself tempted with takeout.
4. 1+1+1 Rule
   If you are unsure with where to start with your meal preps, remember the 1+1+1 rule. Essentially, this just means that you will want to have a protein, a carb, and a fresh produce with every meal. Of course, these portions will change depending on what your goals are, but this is a pretty basic plan to follow.

5. Bulk Buy

Another excuse people use when it comes to meal prepping and eating healthy is that it is just too expensive. Luckily for you, there are ways to save money. When you buy in bulk, it helps lower the price. By doing this, you will be able to cook enough for the week and freeze the rest to be used at a later time.

6. Reflect on Your Goals

When selecting your recipes, they should reflect your goals. As I said before, you will need to balance your complex carbs, your healthy fats, and your proteins. You will want to do the best you can to avoid refined sugars and artificial sweeteners. Below, you will find a basic list to add to your grocery list

Proteins:

Turkey, chicken, steak, ground beef, tuna, eggs, lentils, tofu, pinto beans, black beans, salmon, shrimp, and chickpeas.

Vegetables:

Spinach, collard greens, kale, squash, peppers, carrots, cauliflower, green beans, mushrooms, asparagus, beets, and broccoli.

Carbohydrates:

Whole wheat bread, whole wheat pasta, brown rice, oats, sweet potatoes, and quinoa.

Healthy Fats

Nut butter, avocado oil, olive oil, coconut oil, cashews, olives, avocado, and almonds.

Fruits:

Apples, blueberries, strawberries, raspberries, blackberries, oranges, pineapple, melon, mangoes, and bananas.

Of course, this isn't a complete list. The best part of meal prepping is how customizable it is. All you have to do is take the time to sit down and decide what your goals are. Are you looking to lose weight? Perhaps you would like to gain some weight? No matter what, you can choose the foods you want to consume and go from there!

Meal Prep Pros and Cons

Just like with any diet, meal prepping just isn't for everyone! But, you are here for a reason, right? Below, I will list just some of the pros and cons that come with meal prepping. After, you can decide if this lifestyle would be best for you.

Pros:

1. Free Time
   At this point, you understand that meal prepping is meant to save you time. Indeed, once all of your cooking is done, you will have the rest of your week to do as you please! You will have no excuse to eat unhealthy because it will already be made! By prepping your meals, time will be one less thing you have to worry about.
2. Thoughtful Meals
   The whole point of meal prepping is to eat healthier. By taking the time to sit down and create your meals at the beginning of the week, you are taking the time to put your health first. By planning, you won't have the time or thought to opt for an easier, less healthy meal.
3. Portion Controls
   If you are looking to lose weight, meal prep will be one of your essential goals. Sometimes when people cook their meals, they throw any sense of portion control out the window. When you are meal prepping, you become more aware of portions as only a certain amount of food can fit into your containers in the first place!
4. Decrease Temptation
   We have all been there. Perhaps driving home or laying on the couch, you think about how much easier it would be to order out or drive through somewhere instead of taking the time to cook. I understand it can be incredibly tempting.

However, when you meal prep, it is like a healthier version of takeout!

5. Saving Money
   As I mentioned before, meal prepping is a great way to save money. First off, you can buy in bulk to help lower the price of the foods you are buying. You will also be saving money by not eating out all of the time! Often times, we are not aware of it, but we do spend a lot of money out, just because of the convenience. Why not make your meals more convenient and healthy at the same time!

Cons

1. Exhausting
   Cooking isn't for everyone, I understand that. It can be tiring to spend a few hours in the kitchen cooking up your meals. Meal prepping is going to take time and effort, there is no getting around that. This is just another reason I suggest choosing a day where you can take your time with meal prepping. It will take some time to shop, cook, and clean the dishes after. Who says you need to rush? As long as you anticipate the time needed, there is no need to feel exhausted by meal prepping.
2. Bored
   Eating the same meals during the week can be incredibly boring. This is especially true if you plan a meal and just don't feel like eating that particular food that day. This is why I suggest prepping multiple meals during the week. You will want to choose recipes that you can get excited over. If you feel that you are forcing yourself to eat a meal, there is no way you will stick to the lifestyle. You are in charge of what you are eating and cooking, choose wisely!
3. Portion Control
   There is a popular term circulating society known as HANGRY. You know, that feeling you get when you are just so hungry that you get mad. If you are looking

to lose weight, you may experience this with meal prepping. As you meal prep, you will be focused on making your portions smaller. As a suggestion, I will tell you to decrease your serving sizes slowly. You will need to shrink your stomach so it can get used to smaller portions. If you dive right into it, you will increase your desire to overeat. Avoid this and start slow as I keep suggesting.

Choosing a Plan

We are all here for different reasons. Some are looking to save time, others looking to eat healthier. Whether you are looking to lose weight or gain weight, there are different ways to look at your meal prepping. One way to look at it is to count calories. We suggest planning your meals depending on your macronutrients. This way, you can plan specific foods for your meals without having to count all of those calories. You will want to use an online calculator to decide what your macronutrients will look like. Here is the basic information you will need:

1. Age
2. Sex
3. Height
4. Weight
5. Goal (Fat Loss, Muscle Gain, Maintenance)
6. Activity Level (Light, Moderate, Active)

By using the information above, a calculator can give you the macronutrients to meet your goal. Once this is determined, you can go ahead and choose your meals for the week. As a basic recommended macronutrient ratio, it is recommended to have 35% protein, 25% carbohydrates, and 40% fats. As discussed, these numbers will change depending on your health goals.

Meal Prep Examples:

Breakfast M/W/F: Oat and Jam Muffins

Breakfast T/Thu: Detox Ginger and Peach Smoothie

Lunch M/W/F: Tangy Lemon Thyme Chicken

Lunch T/Thu: Easy Turkey Chili

Dinner M/W/F: Crusted Herb Pork Chops + Garlic Roasted Cauliflower

Dinner M/W/F: Spicy Moroccan Salmon + Cilantro and Lime Cauliflower Rice

Breakfast M/W/F: Oatmeal Carrot Cake Breakfast Bars

Breakfast T/Thu: CPK Smoothie

Lunch M/W/F: Zesty Lime and Cilantro Chicken Tacos

Lunch T/Thu: Spicy Crab Stuffed Cucumber Cups

Dinner M/W/F: Slow Cooker Tomato and Beef Stew

Dinner T/ Thu: Pesto and Tomato Chicken Rolls + Simple Roasted Asparagus

Breakfast M/W/F: Sweet Apple Cider Oatmeal Breakfast

Breakfast T/Thu: Banana and Oat Breakfast Smoothie

Lunch M/W/F: One Pan Cashew and Chicken Stir Fry

Lunch T/Thu: Sweet and Spicy Glazed Sriracha Meatballs + Roasted Butternut Squash

Dinner M/W/F: Grilled Onion and Peppers Tilapia Tacos

Dinner T/Thu: Baked Taco Pie

Breakfast M/W/F: Veggie Eggie Breakfast Muffins

Breakfast T/Thu: Oat and Strawberry Jam Muffins

Lunch M/W/F: Chicken Bruschetta

Lunch T/Thu: Avocado and Spicy Tuna Wrap

Dinner M/W/F: Jerk Caribbean Shrimp + Lemon and Garlic Roasted Broccoli

Dinner M/W/F: Spicy Sausage Spaghetti Squash Ships

As for snacks and desserts, feel free to sprinkle these in as needed. It is important to stick to your calorie goal but also allow yourself a treat every once in a while. If you don't, you run a higher risk of eating more of the bad foods you are craving.

Chapter Two: Breakfast Recipes

Mixed Berry Slow Cooker Breakfast Quinoa

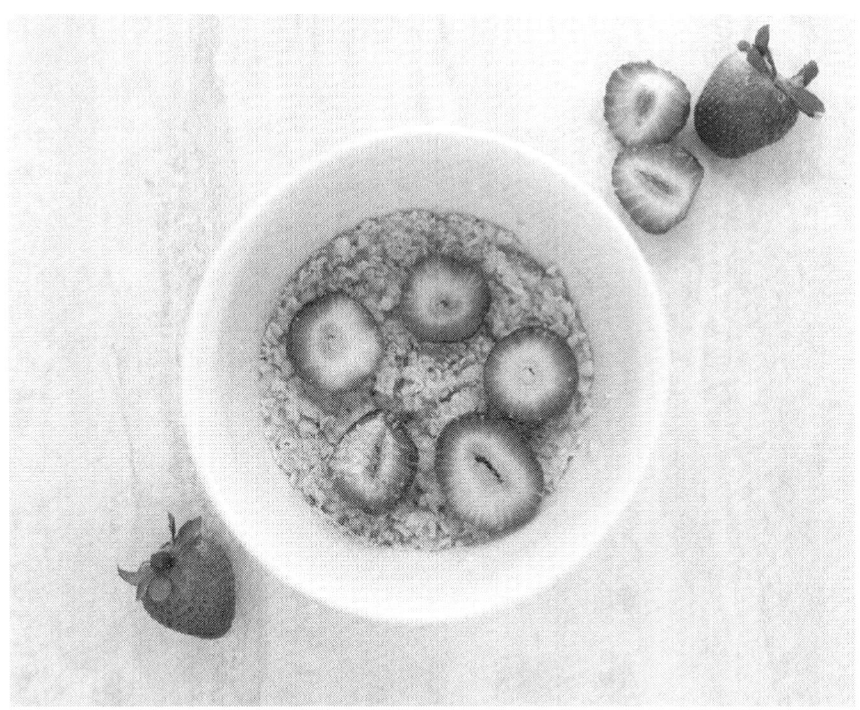

Eight Servings
Serving Size: One Cup
Carbohydrates: 44g
Proteins: 7g
Fats: 3g

Ingredients:

- Vanilla Extract (2 t.)
- Maple Syrup (2 T.)
- Cinnamon (1 t.)
- Salt (.15 t.)
- Mixed Berries (2 C.)
- Quinoa (2 C.)
- Water (4 C.)
- Bananas (2)

Directions:

1. To start off, you will want to take your slow cooker and coat it with your cooking spray of choice. Once it is covered, toss in all of the ingredients from the list above.
2. Once the ingredients have been placed, turn your slow cooker on low and allow this mixture to cook for five to six hours.
3. For additional flavors, add in your favorite nuts or fruit! Spoon a cup into each container and store in the fridge for a quick and easy breakfast.

Veggie Eggie Breakfast Muffins
Twelve Servings
Serving Size: One Muffin
Carbohydrates: 3g
Proteins: 5g
Fats: 5g

Ingredients:

- Arugula (2 C.)
- Red Bell Pepper (1)
- Eggs (8)
- Garlic (2 Cloves)
- Onion (.5)
- Olive Oil (1 T.)
- Parmesan Cheese (.25 C.)
- Salt & Pepper (Pinch)

Directions:

1. You will want to start off by heating your oven to 375 degrees.
2. As your oven heats up, take a muffin tin and spray it with your cooking spray of choice.
3. In a medium pan, begin to heat up your tablespoon of olive oil. When the olive oil begins to sizzle, toss in your onion and garlic and cook for five minutes or so. Once these are cooked, you can also throw in your bell peppers.
4. When all of your vegetables are cooked, chop them up and place into the bottom of each muffin tin.
5. In a bowl, whisk your cheese, arugula, and eggs all together. If desired, you can take this time to season the eggs with salt and pepper.
6. When the egg mixture is ready, go ahead and pour it evenly into each muffin hole. Be sure not to overfill the tins as the eggs will rise slightly during the cooking process.

7. Finally, pop the tin in for about twenty minutes. This should be enough time to cook through.
8. When they are done, allow them to cool and place each egg muffin into a container for an easy to go breakfast muffin.

Oat and Strawberry Jam Muffins
Twelve Servings
Serving Size: One Muffin
Carbohydrates: 21g
Proteins: 5g
Fats: 4g

Ingredients:

- Strawberry Jam (.25 C.)
- Vanilla Extract (1 t.)
- Honey (1 T.)
- Coconut Oil (2 T.)
- Almond Milk (1 C.)
- Eggs (2)
- Stevia (.50 C.)
- Baking Powder (1 T.)
- Oat Flour (.50 C.)
- Whole Wheat Flour (2 C.)

Directions:

1. Start off by heating your oven to 425 degrees.
2. As the oven heats up, take out a small bowl and use a flour sifter to sift through your oat flour, whole wheat flour, and the baking powder.
3. Once this is in place, you will want to toss in your half cup of stevia and mix everything together.
4. In a different bowl, mix together the almond milk, melted coconut oil, eggs, vanilla extract, and the honey.
5. Now, pour the wet ingredients over your dry ingredients and mix everything together.
6. Next, you will want to take a greased muffin tin pan and spoon the batter between each one of the holes.
7. When the muffin tins are filled, go ahead and teaspoon the strawberry jam on top of the batter. Using a toothpick, you will want to swirl the ingredients together. For a lower calorie option, try sugar-free jam in your muffins.

8. Once the muffins are ready, toss them into the oven for twenty minutes. They will be ready when you are able to stick a toothpick in the middle, and it comes out clean.
9. When done, remove muffins from the oven and allow them to cool.

Sweet and Spicy Sweet Potato Hash Browns

Two Servings
Serving Size: .5 C.
Carbohydrates: 30g
Proteins: 3g
Fats: 8g

Ingredients:

- Chili Powder (.15 t.)
- Cinnamon (.15 t.)
- Salt (.50 t.)
- Butter (3 T.)
- Onion (.50 C.)
- Sweet Potatoes (2)
- Black Pepper (Pinch)

Directions:

1. You will want to start off by preparing your sweet potatoes. You can do this by peeling and shredding the sweet potatoes with a grater. Be sure to squeeze any excess water out, as this may mess up the recipe.
2. Once your sweet potato is prepared, take a skillet and begin to melt the butter from the list above. Once the butter is melted, toss in your onion and cook for a total of two minutes. Season the mixture with the chili powder, salt, pepper, and cinnamon.
3. When the onion is cooked through, add in your grated sweet potato. Allow this mixture to cook for five to eight minutes. It is cooked through once it becomes a browned color.
4. When it begins to brown, flip the sweet potato mixture over and be sure to cook the other side for around five minutes or so.

5. Once both sides are cooked, portion the sweet potatoes into your containers and enjoy with a piece of fruit or perhaps an egg muffin from the recipe above!

Oatmeal Carrot Cake Breakfast Bars
Sixteen Servings
Serving Size: One Bar
Carbohydrates: 16g
Proteins: 4g
Fats: 6g

Ingredients:

- Carrots (.50, grated)
- Vanilla Extract (1 t.)
- Maple Syrup (.50 C.)
- Coconut Oil (.25 C.)
- Soy Milk (1 C.)
- Egg (1)
- Nutmeg (.15 t.)
- Cinnamon (2 t.)
- Baking Powder (1 t.)
- Rolled Oats (2.50 C.)

Directions:

1. Start off by heating your oven to 350 degrees.
2. While the oven is heating up, take a bowl and mix together your nutmeg, cinnamon, baking powder, and oats. If desired, you can toss in some salt, but it is not needed.
3. In another bowl, whisk together your coconut oil, maple syrup, vanilla, eggs, and milk.
4. Once both are prepared, you can mix together your wet and dry ingredients in the same bowl.
5. Now that you have your mixture, you can pour it into a greased baking dish.
6. Pop this dish in your heated oven for a total of forty minutes.

7. Remove the dish from the oven, allow to cool, and slice into bars for easy, on the go breakfast bars!

Overnight Oats Blueberry Muffin Style
One Serving
Serving Size: One Jar
Carbohydrates: 41g
Proteins: 14g
Fats: 6g

Ingredients:

- Blueberries (.25 C.)
- Vanilla Extract (1 t.)
- Cinnamon (.15 t.)
- Honey (.50 T.)
- Chia Seeds (1 T.)
- Almond Milk (.33 C.)
- Greek Yogurt (.33 C.)
- Rolled Oats (.33 C.)

Directions:

1. Take a jar or a bowl and place your yogurt, chia seeds, honey, vanilla, cinnamon, and oats all together.
2. Once everything is well combined, cover the jar/bowl with plastic wrap and pop it into the fridge overnight.
3. When you are ready to enjoy your meal, cover with fresh blueberries, and you have a quick and healthy meal!

Sweet Apple Cider Oatmeal Breakfast
Eight Servings
Serving Size: .75 C.
Carbohydrates: 43g
Proteins: 4g
Fats: 10g

Ingredients:

- Cinnamon Sticks (2)
- Maple Syrup (.33 C.)
- Apple Cider (2 C.)
- Apples (6)

Topping Ingredients:

- Allspice (.50 t.)
- Cinnamon (1 t.)
- Vanilla Extract (1 t.)
- Apple Cider Mix (.25 C.)
- Almond Flour (.50 C.) + (2 T.)
- Pecans (.50 C.)
- Rolled Oats (1 C.)

Directions:

1. To begin, you will want to heat your oven to 375 degrees.
2. While this is heating up, go ahead and prep your apples by washing, peeling and slicing them. Once they are done, set them aside in a bowl.
3. Over medium heat, bring a small saucepan with the apple cider, maple syrup, and cinnamon to a boil. Once it is boiling, turn the heat lower and allow this mixture to simmer for around twenty minutes. Now, the liquid should be reduced, and you can pour this mixture over your apples. Be sure to reserve .25 C. of this liquid for later use.
4. In another bowl, mix together your pecans, almond flour, apple cider mixture, cinnamon, salt, allspice, vanilla, and the rolled oats.

5. Now that these are ready, place the apples into a baking dish and sprinkle the above mixture over the top.
6. Pop the dish into your oven for thirty minutes. By the end, your apples should be tender and delicious.
7. Spoon the mixture into ¾ cups into your containers and breakfast will be ready for you when you want it!

CPK Smoothie
Two Servings
Serving Size: 1 C.
Carbohydrates: 41g
Proteins: 8g
Fats: 5g

Ingredients:

- Chia Seeds (2 T.)
- Orange Juice (.25 C.)
- Pineapple (.25 C.)
- Greek Yogurt (.50 C.)
- Banana (1)
- Kiwi (1 C.)
- Spinach (2 C.)

Directions:

1. First, you will want to prepare all of the ingredients from above. Be sure they are washed, peeled, and chopped into smaller pieces.
2. Once this is done, toss them into a blender and blend for thirty seconds or until they are well combined.
3. Divide your smoothie into proper portions and store until ready to be served for a quick and easy breakfast idea.

Banana and Oat Breakfast Smoothie
Two Servings
Serving Size: 1 C.
Carbohydrates: 33g
Proteins: 6g
Fats: 8g

Ingredients:

- Almond Milk (.50 C.)
- Cinnamon (.50 t.)
- Flaxseed Meal (1 T.)
- Banana (1)
- Yogurt (.50 C.)
- Rolled Oats (.33 C.)

Directions:

1. Begin by preparing the banana. Be sure it is washed, peeled, and chopped into smaller pieces.
2. Toss all of the ingredients from the list above into a blender and blend for thirty seconds or until everything is well combined.
3. Separate the smoothie into two servings and breakfast is ready.

Detox Ginger and Peach Smoothie

Two Servings
Serving Size: .50 C.
Carbohydrates: 27g
Proteins: 6g
Fats: .5g

Ingredients:

- Coconut Water (1 C.)
- Stevia (1 Packet)
- Greek Yogurt (.25 C.)
- Ginger (1 T.)
- Banana (.50)
- Peaches (2 C.)
- Spinach (1 C.)

Directions:

1. Take all of the ingredients from the list above and toss them into your blender.
2. Blend for thirty seconds or until everything is well combined. For a thicker smoothie, try adding in ice.
3. Finally, portion out your smoothie and breakfast is ready.

Homemade Nut Bar

Ten Servings
Serving Size: One Bar
Carbohydrates: 18g
Proteins: 5g
Fats: 12g

Ingredients:

- Dark Chocolate Chips (.50 C.)
- Salt (.50 t.)
- Vanilla Extract (.50 t.)
- Honey (2 T.)
- Brown Rice Syrup (.25 C.)
- Flaxseed Meal (1 T.)
- Puffed Rice (.33 C.)
- Walnuts (.50 C.)
- Dry Roasted Peanuts (.50 C.)
- Dry Roasted Almonds (.50 C.)

Directions:

1. Begin by lining a pan with aluminum foil so that it is prepared for this recipe.
2. Now, take a small bowl and mix together the flaxseed meal, puffed rice, and the nuts.
3. In a saucepan, bring the following to a boil: salt, vanilla, honey, and brown rice syrup. Continue to stir this mixture for two minutes or so.
4. When this is done, pour the wet ingredients over the nuts and combine everything.
5. Place this mixture into the bottom of the pan and be sure to spread it out evenly so that there are no gaps.
6. Pop the dish into the fridge and allow it to cool for twenty to thirty minutes or until solid.
7. For a finishing touch, go ahead and melt the chocolate chips. Carefully drizzle the chocolate over the mixture and then cut them into bars.

8. Portion out your bars, and you have an easy to grab breakfast!

Chapter Three: Chicken Recipes

Tangy Lemon Thyme Chicken

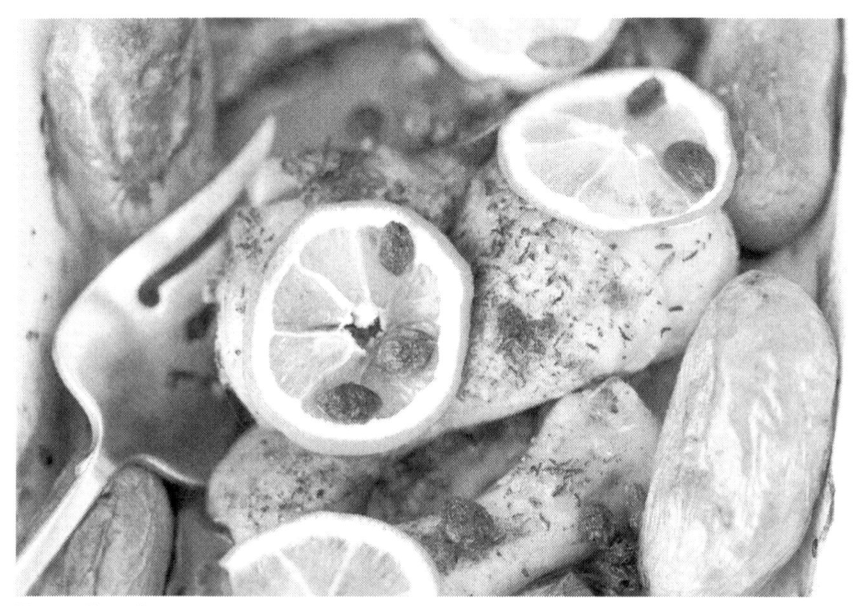

Four Servings
Serving Size: One Chicken Breast
Carbohydrates: 3g
Proteins: 25g
Fats: 4g

Ingredients:

- Thyme (1 T.)
- Salt (1 t.)
- Pepper (.50 t.)
- Lemon (1-Zest)
- Lemons (2-Juice)
- Chicken Breast (4)

Directions:

1. Start out by heating your oven to 375 degrees.

2. While this is warming up, take a small bowl and mix together your lemon zest, lemon juice, salt, pepper, and the thyme.
3. When you are ready, place the chicken breast into the bottom of a baking dish and pour the lemon mixture over the top. Be sure to swirl the dish around to assure the chicken is completely coated.
4. Finally, pop the dish into the oven for forty minutes or so. When it is cooked through, the juices will run clear. Once cooked, remove from the oven, cool, and portion one breast per container. For a well-rounded meal, pair with a favorite veggie.

Chicken Bruschetta
Four Servings
Serving Size: One Chicken Breast and .33 C. of Bruschetta
Carbohydrates: 8g
Proteins: 28g
Fats: 4g

Ingredients:

- Basil (.25 C.)
- Salt (.10 t.)
- Balsamic Vinegar (1 t.)
- Olive Oil (1 t.)
- Red Onion (.50)
- Garlic (1)
- Tomatoes (5)
- Chicken Breast (4)

Directions:

1. Begin by heating your oven to 375 degrees.
2. If you desire, season the chicken breast with salt and pepper before popping it onto a baking sheet. Place the chicken in the oven for about forty minutes.
3. While the chicken bakes, take a small bowl and mix together your basil, balsamic vinegar, olive oil, onion, garlic, and the chopped tomatoes.
4. Finally, remove your chicken from the oven and allow to cool. Portion out your chicken into your containers, and you have a very healthy lunch or dinner.

Herb and Balsamic Maple Chicken

Four Servings
Serving Size: One Chicken Breast
Carbohydrates: 10g
Proteins: 27g
Fats: 10g

Ingredients:

- Olive Oil (2 T.)
- Cayenne Pepper (1 t.)
- Garlic (2)
- Dijon Mustard (1 T.)
- Maple Syrup (2 T.)
- Balsamic Vinegar (.25 C.)
- Chicken Breast (4)
- Salt (.50 t.)
- Pepper (.50 t.)

Directions:

1. To begin, you will be making your marinate. This will take thirty minutes, but for better flavor, it is suggested to soak the chicken overnight. Create this mixture by blending the maple syrup, mustard, balsamic vinegar, thyme, salt, pepper, cayenne, and garlic all together. Once this is done, pour over your chicken and allow to oak.
2. When the chicken is seasoned as desired, place in a skillet over medium heat with some olive oil. Cook each side of the chicken for eight minutes or until it is cooked through. Once one side turns a golden-brown color, cook the other side for another eight minutes.
3. Portion out the chicken to your containers and eat with a delicious vegetable for a well-rounded meal.

Quinoa Chicken Fajita Soup in Slow Cooker
Six Servings
Serving Size: 1.50 C.
Carbohydrates: 50g
Proteins: 30g
Fats: 5g

Ingredients:

- Salt (2 t.)
- Paprika (2 t.)
- Cumin (1 T.)
- Chili Powder (1.50 T.)
- Corn (1 C.)
- Black Beans (1 Can)
- Green Chiles (1 Can)
- Diced Tomatoes (1 Can)
- Lime (1-Juice)
- Low-sodium Chicken Broth (4 C.)
- Garlic (3)
- Onion (1)
- Bell Peppers (3)
- Quinoa (1 C.)
- Chicken Breast (1.50 Lbs.)

Directions:

1. The best part of the slow cooker is being able to toss all of the ingredients from above into it and forgetting about it. If you need a quick meal, toss all of the ingredients on high for four hours. For a slower cook, put the mixture on a low heat for eight hours.
2. Once the chicken is cooked through, turn the heat off and allow to cool. You will want to take two forks and gently shred the chicken. If you want, go ahead and season with salt and pepper to taste.

3. Finally, portion out your soup and you have a quick meal for lunch or dinner.

One Pan Tangy Rosemary Chicken with Potatoes
Four Servings
Serving Size: One Chicken Breast, .50 C. Potatoes, .25 C. Green Beans
Carbohydrates: 26g
Proteins: 39g
Fats: 3g

Ingredients:

- Green Beans (1 Lb.)
- Red Potatoes (3 C.)
- Chicken Breast (4)
- Black Pepper (1 t.)
- Salt (1 t.)
- Thyme (1 T.)
- Rosemary (1 T.)
- Garlic (2)
- Lemon (1-Zest)
- Lemon Juice (1 T.)
- Olive Oil (3 T.)

Directions:

1. Start off this recipe by heating your oven to 400 degrees.
2. While this warms up, take a small bowl and mix together the olive oil, lemon zest, lemon juice, thyme, pepper, salt, and the rosemary.
3. In a different bowl, mix together the baby potatoes with a tablespoon of olive oil. If you would like, you can also add some salt and pepper to this recipe as desired.
4. Now that these are ready, take a large baking dish and arrange your chicken and green beans on it. Once in place, also put the potatoes on the sheet.

5. Finally, drizzle the mixture from above and be sure all of the ingredients are evenly coated.
6. When you are ready, toss the sheet into the oven for thirty minutes or so. When you pull it out, the chicken should be cooked through, and the green beans will be crisp.
7. Once cooked, portion out the ingredients from above and enjoy!

One Pan Cashew and Chicken Stir Fry
Six Servings
Serving Size: 1 C.
Carbohydrates: 18g
Proteins: 21g
Fats: 3g

Ingredients:

- Unsalted Cashews (.33 C.)
- Green Onions (4)
- Carrots (.50 C.)
- Sugar Snap Peas (1 C.)
- Red Bell Pepper (1)
- Broccoli (2 C.)
- Chicken Breast (1 Lb.)
- Olive Oil (1 T.)
- Garlic (3)

Sauce:

- Water (3 T.)
- Ginger (1 T.)
- Sesame Oil (1 t.)
- Honey (2 T.)
- Peanut Butter (3 T.)
- Soy Sauce (4 T.)

Directions:

1. To begin, you will start by making the sauce for this recipe. You can do so by taking a small bowl and mixing together the water, ginger, sesame oil, honey, peanut butter, and the soy sauce. You can add more water for a thinner sauce.
2. Once this is done, begin to heat the olive oil in a medium size pan over medium heat. Once the olive oil is sizzling, add in your chicken and cook on either side. This should

take ten minutes or so. Once cooked through, season with garlic, salt, and the pepper.

3. When you feel the chicken is cooked through, you can add in the broccoli, snap peas, bell pepper, and carrots and allow them to cook. This should take an extra five minutes.
4. Now that all of your ingredients are cooked, drizzle the sauce over and be sure to coat everything evenly.
5. Finally, add in your cashews as a final touch. Portion out the meal, and you have a delicious lunch or dinner for the week!

Zesty Lime and Cilantro Chicken Tacos

Five Servings
Serving Size: Two Tacos
Carbohydrates: 60g
Proteins: 36g
Fats: 20g

Ingredients:

- Whole Wheat Tortillas (10)
- Chicken (1.50 Lbs.)

Marinade:

- Cilantro (2 T.)
- Honey (.50 t.)
- Garlic (2)
- Olive Oil (1 T.)
- Lime (2-Juice)
- Lime (1-Zest)

Topping Coleslaw:

- Honey (1 t.)
- Olive Oil (1 T.)
- Lime (2)
- Green Onion (.50 C.)
- Cilantro (.50 C.)
- Carrots (1 C.)
- Red Cabbage (1 C.)
- Green Cabbage (2 C.)

Directions:

1. Begin by making your marinade. You will do this by mixing together the cilantro, honey, garlic, olive oil, lime zest, and lime juice. When it is combined, toss in your chicken and allow it to soak for four hours or best, overnight.

2. In the meantime, you can make the coleslaw by first, shredding the cabbages and carrots. Mix these together with the olive oil, honey, and lime juice.
3. Once the chicken is seasoned properly, take a medium pan over medium heat and cook the chicken for five minutes on either side. Be sure that the chicken is cooked through.
4. When you are ready to prep your meals, place the chicken into the tortillas and top with the coleslaw.

Sweet Hawaiian Pineapple and Chicken Kabobs
Five Servings
Serving Size: 2 Skewers
Carbohydrates: 21g
Proteins: 26g
Fats: .2g

Ingredients:

- Pineapple (3 C.)
- Onion (1)
- Bell Peppers (3)
- Chicken Breast (1.25 Lbs.)

Marinade:

- Garlic (2)
- Grated Ginger (2 t.)
- Hot Chili Paste (1 T.)
- Olive Oil (1 T.)
- Honey (1 T.)
- Soy Sauce (.25 C.)
- Pineapple Juice (.25 C.)

Directions:

1. Start off by making your marinade for the chicken. Do this by taking the ingredients from above and mixing it all together in a small to a medium-sized bowl. When this is done, pour it over your chicken and allow it to soak for at least an hour. When pouring over your chicken, save .25 C. of the marinade for later use.
2. Once the chicken is ready, prepare the bell peppers, pineapple, and onion by cutting them into smaller chunks. When this is done, go ahead and place a skewer through the ingredients to create your kabobs.
3. When this is done, place the kebobs on the grill or oven for four to five minutes on each side. If you want, brush the

marinade you reserved from earlier over the kabobs to keep them moist.

4. Finally, portion out the skewers and try with a delicious quinoa side.

Pesto and Tomato Chicken Rolls
Six Servings
Serving Size: One Chicken Roll
Carbohydrates: 14g
Proteins: 42g
Fats: 17g

Ingredients:

- Crushed Tomatoes (1 Can)
- Mozzarella Cheese (.50 C.)
- Egg (1)
- Shredded Cheese (.25 C.)
- Garlic Powder (.50 t.)
- Oregano (1 t.)
- Flaxseed Meal (2 T.)
- Whole Wheat Panko Breadcrumbs (.50 C.)
- Chicken Breast (6)
- Salt (.50 t.)
- Pepper (.50 t.)

Pesto Sauce:

- Salt (.50 t.)
- Pepper (.50 t.)
- Basil Leaves (1 C.)
- Parmesan Cheese (1 C.)
- Garlic (3)
- Tomatoes (1 Jar)

Directions:

1. To begin, you will want to heat your oven to 375 degrees.
2. Now, as this heats up, make the pesto sauce. You will do this by adding the pesto sauce ingredients from the list above and pulsing in a food processor. Once this is done, put the sauce to the side.

3. Now, you will need a meat tenderizer to flatten your chicken breast to about .25 in. thick. Once this is done, season it with salt and pepper and spread your fresh made pesto onto the chicken. For a final touch, sprinkle in the shredded cheese and roll the chicken up. You can secure this with the help of a toothpick.
4. In a small bowl, add in the garlic powder, oregano, flaxseed meal, and breadcrumbs.
5. In another bowl, mix together the egg with a couple tablespoons of water.
6. When you are ready, dip the rolled chicken into the egg mixture and coat the chicken with the breadcrumbs.
7. Once this is complete, place the chicken rolls onto a sheet and cook for thirty minutes in the oven.
8. Finally, remove the chicken, place mozzarella over the top and cook for another five minutes to allow the cheese to melt.
9. Portion out the chicken rolls into your containers, and you have a delicious, ready to go meal.

Ginger and Turmeric Grilled Chicken

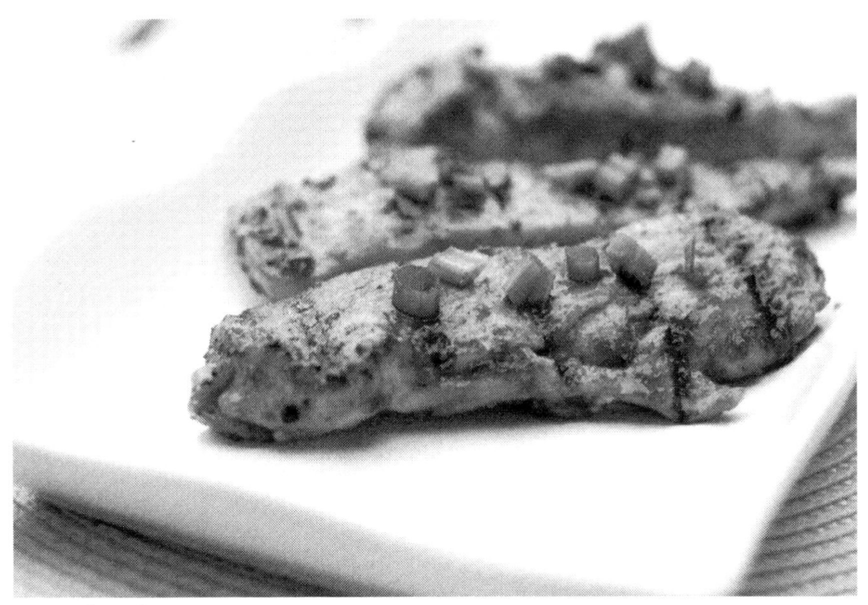

Four Servings
Serving Size: One Chicken Breast
Carbohydrates: 3g
Proteins: 48g
Fats: 10g

Ingredients:

- Lime Juice (1 T.)
- Salt (.50 t.)
- Pepper (.50 t.)
- Cumin (.50 t.)
- Coriander (1 t.)
- Ginger (1 T.)
- Turmeric (1 t.)
- Garlic (2)
- Olive Oil (1 T.)
- Coconut Milk (.50 Can)
- Chicken Breast (4)

Directions:

1. Begin by mixing together your marinade. Do this by taking a small bowl and mixing together the salt, pepper, lime juice, coriander, ginger, turmeric, garlic, olive oil, and coconut milk.
2. Pour this mixture over the chicken and allow it to marinade for at least one hour. If you have the time, allow this to soak overnight for maximum flavor.
3. When the chicken is ready, place it in a medium pan over medium heat and cook for five or six minutes on either side.
4. For extra flavor, squeeze some fresh lime juice over the chicken.
5. Portion the chicken out and enjoy with your favorite vegetable or rice.

Thin Chicken Pot Pie
Five Serving
Serving Size: One Pie
Carbohydrates: 36g
Proteins: 24g
Fats: 4g

Ingredients:

- Reduced-fat Biscuits (1 Can)
- Pepper (.25 t.)
- Salt (1 t.)
- Green Onions (4)
- Mixed Frozen Vegetables (1 Package)
- Chicken Breast (2 C.)
- Thyme (1 t.)
- Poultry Seasoning (1 t.)
- All-purpose Flour (3 T.)
- Fat-free Chicken Broth (1 C.)
- Half and Half (1 C.)

Directions:

1. Start off by heating your oven to 425 degrees.
2. While this is heating up, you will want to bring the following ingredients to a boil: thyme, poultry seasoning, flour, chicken broth, and the half and half. Once it is boiling, reduce the heat and allow the ingredients to simmer for about four minutes.
3. Once this mixture becomes thick, remove it from the heat and mix in the salt, pepper, green onion, veggies, and chicken.
4. Next, roll out your biscuits and put them into greased muffin tins.
5. Place the biscuit and fill the cup with the chicken filling. Once it is filled, cover up the cups and pierce holes into the top.
6. Pop these into the oven for twelve to fifteen minutes.

7. Remove from oven once the biscuits are golden and they are ready to enjoy!

Chapter Four: Red Meat Recipes

Crusted Herb Pork Chops

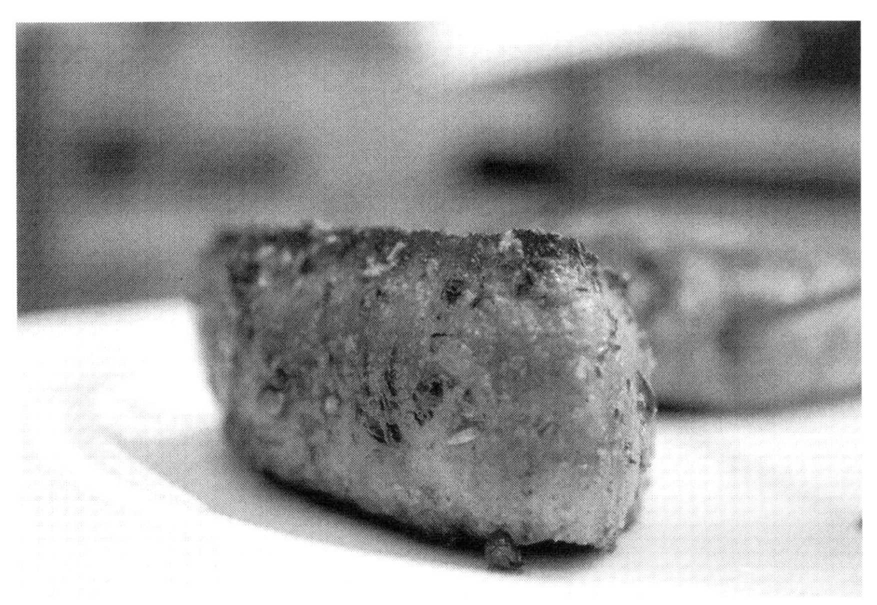

Four Servings
Serving Size: One Pork Chop
Carbohydrates: 5g
Proteins: 25g
Fats: 10g

Ingredients:

- Olive Oil (1 T.)
- Pepper (.50 t.)
- Salt (.50 t.)
- Parsley (1 T.)
- Thyme (1 T.)
- Panko Breadcrumbs (.50 C.)
- Dijon Mustard (2 T.)
- Pork Chops (4)

Directions:

1. Begin by heating your oven to 450 degrees.

2. Next, you will prep your pork chops by rubbing them with the Dijon mustard.
3. In a small bowl, combine the salt, pepper, parsley, thyme, and panko breadcrumbs. For a healthier version, try to get whole wheat breadcrumbs.
4. When you are ready, dip the mustard covered pork chops into the breadcrumbs. Be sure that they are coated evenly.
5. Once they are ready, go ahead and heat a large skillet over medium heat and put your olive oil in. Sauté the chop for two or three minutes on each side before popping it into the oven.
6. Keep the pork chops in the oven for eight to ten minutes before removing and allowing to cool. Portion into your containers and serve with your favorite side.

Spicy Sausage Spaghetti Squash Ships
Four Servings
Serving Size: One Boat
Carbohydrates: 17g
Proteins: 22g
Fats: 14g

Ingredients:

- Basil (2 T.)
- Mozzarella Cheese (.50 C.)
- Pepper (.50 t.)
- Salt (.50 t.)
- Half and Half (.25 C.)
- Tomatoes (1 Can)
- Chicken Broth (1 C.)
- Turkey Sausage (1 Lb.)
- Garlic (1)
- Onion (1)
- Olive Oil (1 T.)
- Spaghetti Squash (2)

Directions:

1. To start, you will be heating your oven to 350 degrees.
2. While this heats up, it is time to prepare your squash. Do this by cutting it down the middle and removing the seeds. Once you have done this, go ahead and place on a baking sheet and stick in the oven for forty-five minutes.
3. As the squash cooks, bring the tablespoon of olive oil to a sizzle in a skillet over medium heat. Once it is, add in the onion, garlic, and turkey sausage until it is cooked through. Once this happens, you can add in the salt, pepper, half and half, tomatoes and the chicken broth.
4. Now that the squash is cooked, remove from the oven and allow it to cool for a bit. When you can, shred the squash with two forks and remove into a bowl. In this bowl, mix

together the spaghetti squash with the cheese and put it back into the bowl with the other mixture.

5. If desired, top with more cheese and pop it into the oven to melt the cheese. Top with basil and your meal is ready!

Sweet and Spicy Glazed Sriracha Meatballs
Eight Servings
Serving Size: Five Meatballs
Carbohydrates: 19g
Proteins: 27g
Fats: 11

Ingredients:

- Black Pepper (.50 t.)
- Salt (.50 t.)
- Garlic Powder (.50 t.)
- Green Onion (.25 C.)
- Eggs (2)
- Panko Breadcrumbs (1 C.)
- Ground Turkey (2 Lbs.)

Sauce:

- Toasted Sesame Oil (.50 t.)
- Garlic (3)
- Ginger (1 T.)
- Honey (3 T.)
- Rice Vinegar (3 T.)
- Soy Sauce (3 T.)
- Sriracha (.25 C.)

Directions:

1. Start by heating your oven to 375 degrees.
2. In a bowl, mix together the salt, pepper, garlic powder, green onion, breadcrumbs, and the turkey. Once this is done, you will want to shape the mix into balls around 1 inch or so. This recipe should make about 40 balls.
3. When the balls are made, place them on a greased baking sheet and pop them in the oven for twenty-five minutes or until they turn a nice, brown color.

4. While these are cooking, you will want to make the sauce. Take a small bowl and combine the ingredients from the list above. Place it in a small pan over a medium heat and allow it to simmer for ten minutes.
5. Finally, toss the balls in the sauce, portion into your containers, and serve with vegetables or even brown rice!

Easy Turkey Chili

Eight Servings
Serving Size: One Cup
Carbohydrates: 26g
Proteins: 35g
Fats: 4g

Ingredients:

- Cayenne Pepper (.10 t.)
- Oregano (2 t.)
- Chili Powder (3 T.)
- Stevia (1 Packet)
- Pepper (.50 t.)
- Salt (.50 t.)
- Jalapenos (2)
- Bell Peppers (2)
- Kidney Beans (1 Can)
- Hot Sauce (.50 t.)
- Tomato Paste (3 T.)
- Diced Tomatoes (1 Can)
- Crushed Tomatoes (1 Can)
- Olive Oil (1 T.)
- Garlic (5)
- Onion (1)
- Ground Turkey (2 Lbs.)

Directions:

1. To start, you will want to place your olive oil, onion, and garlic into a large pot and allow this to cook for a couple of minutes. Once you can smell the garlic, add in your turkey and cook it for ten minutes or until it is brown.
2. Finally, toss in the rest of the ingredients from the list above. Be sure to stir everything together so it becomes well combined. Allow this to cook for an hour over a low heat and then portion into your containers.

Slow Cooker Tomato and Beef Stew
Eight Servings
Serving Size: One and a Half Cups
Carbohydrates: 25g
Proteins: 28g
Fats: 14g

Ingredients:

- Bay Leaf (1)
- Rosemary (2 t.)
- Thyme (1 T.)
- Garlic Powder (2 t.)
- Pepper (.50 t.)
- Salt (1 t.)
- Potatoes (1 lb.)
- Peas (1 C.)
- Celery (3)
- Carrots (3)
- Onion (1)
- Worcestershire Sauce (1 T.)
- Beef Broth (2 C.)
- Tomato Paste (1 Can)
- Stewed Tomatoes (1 Can)
- Stew Beef (2 Lbs.)
- Olive Oil (1 T.)

Directions:

1. This recipe can be made in a number of different ways including instant pot, slow cooker, and even over your stove top.
2. If you are using a slow cooker, pop all of the ingredients from the list above into it and cook on low for about eight hours. As for stovetop, you will want to cook the meat first and then cook in a large pot with the rest of the ingredients for about three hours over a low heat.

3. Either way, allow the meat to cook through, portion into your containers, and enjoy!

Slow Cooked BBQ Pulled Pork
Eight Servings
Serving Size: 1 C.
Carbohydrates: 50g
Proteins: 22g
Fats: 5g

Ingredients:

- Whole Wheat Hamburger Buns (8)
- BBQ Sauce (1 Bottle)
- Diet Root Beer (1 Can)
- Pork Tenderloin (2 Lbs.)

Directions:

1. For a quick dinner, this is the perfect recipe for a delicious dinner.
2. First, pop the tenderloin onto the bottom of the slow cooker. Once in place, pour the diet root beer and BBQ sauce over the top.
3. Cook the tenderloin on low for about seven hours.
4. Once this time is up, shred the tenderloin and serve with your favorite vegetable.

Creamy Slow Cooked Pot Roast

Twelve Servings
Serving Size: 1 C.
Carbohydrates: 5g
Proteins: 46g
Fats: 24g

Ingredients:

- Pot Roast (5.50 Lbs.)
- Water (1.25 C.)
- Dry Onion Soup Mix (1 Packet)
- Cream of Mushroom Soup (2 Cans)

Directions:

1. Begin by placing the mushroom soup, water, and onion soup mix into the bottom of your slow cooker.
2. Gently place the pot roast over the mixture and spoon it over the top. Be sure that it is covered completely before placing the lid on.
3. For a quicker cook, put the roast on high for four hours. For a slower cook, nine hours on low.
4. In the end, turn off the heat, portion out the roast into your containers and serve with a favorite vegetable recipe.

Baked Taco Pie
Eight Servings
Serving Size: 1 Square
Carbohydrates: 37g
Proteins: 20g
Fats: 19g

Ingredients:

- Corn Chips (1 C.)
- Corn (.50 C.)
- Olive Oil (1 T.)
- Honey (1 T.)
- Egg (1)
- Milk (.33 C.)
- Corn Bread Mix (1 Package)
- Black Beans (1 Can)
- Salsa (1 C.)
- Taco Seasoning (1 Packet)
- Ground Beef (1 Lb.)

Directions:

1. Start off by heating your oven to 350 degrees.
2. While this warms up, you will want to take the time to cook the ground beef. Place it in a skillet over medium heat. Once it is browned, toss in the taco seasoning, salsa, and black beans. Cook for several more minutes and then remove from the heat.
3. Next, take a small bowl and mix together the olive oil, honey, egg, milk, and cornbread mix. Once it is in a smooth consistency, pour into the bottom of a casserole dish.
4. Now, layer your ground beef and sprinkle the corn chips over the top.
5. Pop the whole dish into the oven and cook for thirty-five minutes. Once it is cooked through, remove and cut into

eight different pieces. Portion and place in containers for an easy lunch or dinner on the go.

Easy Baked Beef Lasagna

Twelve Servings
Serving Size: 1 C.
Carbohydrates: 37g
Proteins: 30g
Fats: 22g

Ingredients:

- Parmesan Cheese (.75 C.)
- Mozzarella Cheese (.75 Lbs.)
- Salt (.50 t.)
- Egg (1)
- Ricotta Cheese (16 Oz.)
- Lasagna Noodles (12)
- Parsley (.25 t.)
- Italian Seasoning (1 t.)
- Fennel Seeds (.50 t.)
- Basil Leaves (1.50 t.)
- Sugar (2 T.)
- Water (.50 C.)
- Tomato Sauce (2 Cans)
- Tomato Paste (2 Cans)
- Crushed Tomatoes (1 Can)
- Garlic (2)
- Onion (.50 C.)
- Ground Beef (.75 Lbs.)

Directions:

1. To begin, take a medium skillet and begin to heat it over a medium heat. Once warm, begin to cook the ground beef until it turns brown.
2. Once the beef is cooked, add in the tomato paste, tomato sauce, and the crushed tomatoes along with the water.

3. When everything is boiling, you can use this time to toss in a tablespoon of salt, pepper, parsley, fennel seeds, basil, and sugar.
4. Put a lid on the skillet and lower the heat. Allow this to cook for about an hour or so in a simmer.
5. While this is simmering, bring a pot of water to a boil over high heat. Once the water is boiling, you can toss in the lasagna noodles and cook for ten minutes or so. Once they are done, drain and set to the side.
6. In another bowl, combine the egg, parsley, salt, and ricotta cheese all together.
7. When these two steps are done, bring your oven to 375 degrees.
8. In a baking dish, begin to arrange your lasagna. You will do this by layering the meat sauce on the bottom of the dish followed by a layer of ricotta cheese, topped by some mozzarella cheese. Continue this until the baking dish is ¾ full.
9. Pop the whole baking dish into the oven once you have covered it with tin foil. Cook everything for twenty-five minutes before removing from the oven.
10. Once cool, portion into containers and enjoy your healthy meal!

Simple Meatloaf Dinner

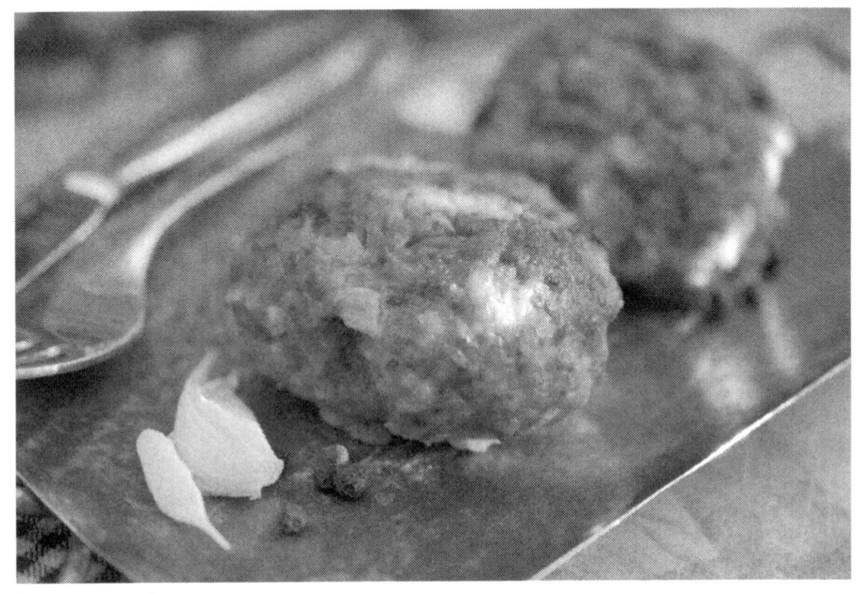

Eight Servings
Serving Size: 1 C.
Carbohydrates: 19g
Proteins: 19g
Fats: 25g

Ingredients:

- Ketchup (.33 C.)
- Mustard (2 T.)
- Brown Sugar (2 T.)
- Salt (.50 t.)
- Pepper (.50 t.)
- Bread Crumbs (1 C.)
- Milk (1 C.)
- Onion (1)
- Egg (1)
- Ground Beef (1.50 Lbs.)

Directions:

1. Start off by heating your oven to 350 degrees.

2. In a mixing bowl, combine the bread crumbs, milk, egg, onion, and the ground beef. Be sure to combine it well so all of the ingredients are well blended.
3. Place this mixture into a baking dish and set to the side.
4. In another bowl, mix together the mustard, ketchup, and brown sugar. Once this is well blended, gently pour it over the meatloaf.
5. Finally, pop the meatloaf into the oven for about an hour or until the beef is cooked through.
6. Cut the meatloaf into twelve slices and portion out according to your needs.

Chapter Five: Seafood Recipes

Grilled Onion and Peppers Tilapia Tacos

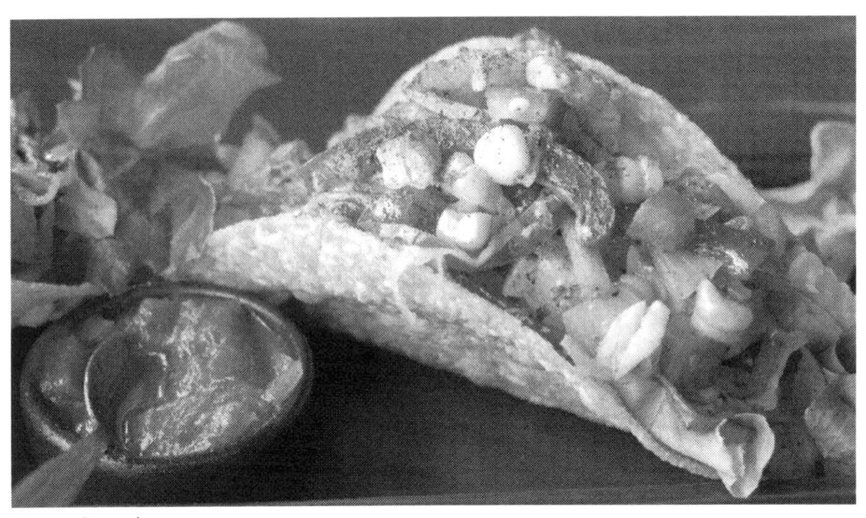

Four Servings
Serving Size: Two Tacos
Carbohydrates: 32g
Proteins: 33g
Fats: 5g

Ingredients:

- Lime (1)
- Jalapeno Pepper (1)
- Corn Tortillas (8)
- Tilapia (4)
- Black Pepper (.50 t.)
- Salt (.50 t.)
- Sweet Bell Peppers (3)
- Onion (2)

Directions:

1. This recipe is recommended to be cooked on the grill for maximum taste but can be done over the stove top as well. To start, you will be cooking the bell peppers and onions

over medium heat. This should take ten to fifteen minutes. Season them with salt and pepper to taste.

2. Once the vegetables are cooked through, season your fish and cook in a pan for around three minutes on each side. Once the fish is cooked through, it will become flakey.
3. Finally, assemble the tacos by placing fish, onion mix, and jalapeno slices into the tortillas. If desired, serve with a slice of lime for some extra flavor.

Spicy Crab Stuffed Cucumber Cups
Six Servings
Serving Size: 3 Cups
Carbohydrates: 5g
Proteins: 9g
Fats: 2g

Ingredients:

- Green Onion (1 T.)
- Black Pepper (.50 t.)
- Salt (.50 t.)
- Crab Meat (.75 C.)
- Cream Cheese (.25 C.)
- Sour Cream (.25 C.)
- Cucumbers (3)
- Paprika (Optional)

Directions:

1. Begin by prepping your cucumbers. You can do this by washing, peeling, and cutting them into two-inch slices.
2. If you have a melon baller, scoop out a hole in the center of each cucumber piece. Once this is done, you can set the cucumber aside.
3. In a small bowl, blend the sour cream and cream cheese together. Once they are smooth, add in the rest of the ingredients.
4. Spoon in the crab mixture into the cucumber cups, and they are ready to be served. For some extra flavor, try sprinkling paprika over the tops!

Spicy Cilantro Shrimp
Four Servings
Serving Size: Six Ounces
Carbohydrates: .5g
Proteins: 35g
Fats: 3g

Ingredients:

- Shrimp (2 Lbs.)
- Cinnamon (.10 t.)
- Cayenne Pepper (.10 t.)
- Curry Powder (.10 t.)
- Ground Cumin (.50 t.)
- Paprika (1 t.)
- Salt (.75 t.)
- Cilantro (Pinch)
- Lime (Optional)

Directions:

1. Begin by making the seasoning for your shrimp. Do this by taking a small bowl and combining the cinnamon, cayenne pepper, curry powder, cumin, paprika, and salt.
2. If you are to cook your shrimp on the grill, it is suggested to skewer the shrimp after seasoning them and cooking them for a minute or two over high heat.
3. As for pan frying, bring olive oil to a sizzle over medium heat and cook the shrimp on both sides for five minutes.
4. For some extra flavor, squeeze the juice of a lime over the top and finish with some fresh chopped cilantro. Portion into containers and you will have a delicious dinner waiting for you.

Roasted Shrimp with Lemon Spaghetti Squash
Four Servings
Serving Size: Two Cups of Spaghetti Squash and Five Shrimp
Carbohydrates: 26g
Proteins: 10g
Fats: 11g

Ingredients:

- Parsley (2 T.)
- Greek Yogurt (.25 C.)
- Red Pepper Flakes (.25 t.)
- Dijon Mustard (1 t.)
- White Wine (.50 C.)
- Lemon Zest (1 t.)
- Garlic (3)
- Salt (.50 t.)
- Pepper (.50 t.)
- Butter (2 T.)
- Olive Oil (1 T.)
- Shrimp (12 Oz.)
- Spaghetti Squash (2)

Directions:

1. Begin by heating your oven to 350 degrees.
2. While the oven heats up, begin to prepare your squash by cutting it down the middle, removing the seeds, and popping it onto a lightly greased baking sheet. You will place the squash in the oven for about forty-five minutes.
3. While the squash cooks, you will want to cook your shrimp in a large skillet over medium heat. Season with salt and pepper to taste and add garlic. This should take four to five minutes to cook the shrimp on either side.
4. Once the shrimp is mostly cooked through, add in the red pepper flakes, Dijon mustard, white wine, lemon zest, and lemon juice, bring this to a boil and then reduce the heat. You will allow this to simmer until the squash is cooked.

5. When the squash is tender, remove from the oven and scrape out the insides.
6. Take the insides, mix together with the sauce and the Greek yogurt. Blend it all together and then scoop back into the squash shell for a delicious meal.

Avocado and Spicy Tuna Wraps
Four Servings
Serving Size: One Wrap
Carbohydrates: 29g
Proteins: 18g
Fats: 2g

Ingredients:

- Whole Wheat Tortillas (4)
- Carrots (1 C.)
- Lettuce (2 C.)
- Salt (.50 t.)
- Pepper (.50 t.)
- Cilantro (1 T.)
- Green Onion (2)
- Onion (2 T.)
- Celery (3 T.)
- Dijon Mustard (1 T.)
- Sriracha (2 T.)
- Avocado (1)
- Tuna (2 Cans)

Directions:

1. In a small bowl, combine the tuna and avocado.
2. Once this is done, you will want to stir in the rest of the ingredients. Use salt and pepper to desired taste.
3. Once this is done, place the mixture into each tortilla wrap and top with the lettuce and carrots. Roll the wraps up tightly, and you have a quick and easy lunch or dinner.

Jerk Caribbean Shrimp
Four Servings
Serving Size: 1 Cup
Carbohydrates: 36g
Proteins: 24g
Fats: 13g

Ingredients:

- Jalapeno (1 T.)
- Green Onion (2 T.)
- Soy Sauce (1 T.)
- Brown Sugar (1 Packet)
- Orange Juice (2 T.)
- Red Wine Vinegar (2 T.)
- Olive Oil (2 T.)
- Shrimp (10 Oz.)

Seasoning:

- Salt (.10 t.)
- Cayenne Pepper (.10 t.)
- Nutmeg (.10 t.)
- Allspice (.10 t.)
- Paprika (.50 t.)
- Thyme (.25 t.)
- Onion Powder (.25 t.)
- Garlic Powder (.50 t.)

Directions:

1. You will begin by making the marinade for the shrimp. You will do this by taking a small bowl and mixing together the following: seasonings, orange juice, red wine vinegar, soy sauce, green onion, brown sugar, jalapeno, and the olive oil. Once this is well blended, add in your shrimp and allow this to soak for about thirty minutes.

2. Place the shrimp on skewers and cook over a medium heat for five or six minutes on either side.
3. Serve the shrimp with your favorite rice or vegetable for a complete and healthy meal.

One Sheet Soy and Ginger Glazed Salmon

Four Servings

Serving Size: One Fillet of Salmon with Half Cup of Carrots and Fourth Cup of Green Beans

Carbohydrates: 25g

Proteins: 48g

Fats: 12g

Ingredients:

- Salt (.50 t.)
- Pepper (.50 t.)
- Olive Oil (1 T.)
- Carrots (2 C.)
- Green Beans (1 Lb.)
- Salmon Fillets (4)

Sauce:

- Green Onions (1 T.)
- Garlic (2)
- Ginger (1 T.)
- Honey (1 T.)
- Sweet Chili Sauce (2 T.)
- Soy Sauce (.25 C.)

Directions:

1. Before you begin cooking, bring your oven to 400 degrees.
2. On a baking sheet, place your green beans, carrots, and salmon skin side down. Drizzle all of the above ingredients with the olive oil and salt and pepper to taste.
3. Take a small bowl and mix together the green onion, garlic, ginger, honey, chili sauce, and the soy sauce. Once this is smooth, spoon it over the salmon and pop the whole pan into the oven.
4. Cook the pan for ten minutes and then turn on the broiler for three minutes so that the salmon comes out crisp.

5. Portion out your meal and dinner will be all ready for you!

Crusted Hummus Salmon

Four Servings
Serving Size: One Salmon Fillet
Carbohydrates: 14g
Proteins: 48g
Fats: 27g

Ingredients:

- Honey (2 t.)
- Dijon Mustard (1.50 t.)
- Butter (.25 C.)
- Thyme (2 t.)
- Parmesan Cheese (.25 C.)
- Panko Breadcrumbs (.50 C.)
- Hummus (.25 C.)
- Salmon Fillets (4)
- Salt (.50 t.)
- Pepper (.50 t.)

Directions:

1. To begin, heat your oven to 375 degrees.
2. Place the salmon fillets onto a baking sheet and season them with salt and pepper to taste. Once this is done, you can spoon a thin layer of hummus over the top of them.
3. In a small bowl, mix together the butter, honey, Dijon mustard, panko bread crumbs, thyme, and parmesan cheese. Once this is well combined, you can go ahead and press it onto each salmon fillet.
4. Bake these for twenty minutes or until the fish becomes flaky. Portion and go!

Crab Cake Baked Balls

Eight Servings
Serving Size: Three Balls
Carbohydrates: 12g
Proteins: 13g
Fats: 1g

Ingredients:

- Black Pepper (.10 t.)
- Salt (.10 t.)
- Panko Breadcrumbs (1 C.)
- Crab Meat (1 Lb.)
- Old Bay Seasoning (1.50 t.)
- Green Onions (2)
- Lemon Juice (2 t.)
- Sriracha (.25 t.)
- Dijon Mustard (1 T.)
- Greek Yogurt (.25 C.)
- Egg (1)

Directions:

1. Start by heating your oven to 350 degrees.
2. While this warms up, take a bowl and mix together the old bay seasoning, lemon juice, green onion, egg, yogurt, and Sriracha. Once this is well combined, you can also add in the crab meat.
3. With this mixture, form one inch balls and place them on a greased sheet. You should be able to make about twenty-four balls with this mixture. Once this is done, pop them into the fridge for thirty minutes.
4. Finally, pop the balls into the oven for thirty minutes. When they are done, they should be a nice golden color. For even crispier balls, try putting them in the broiler for another five minutes.

5. Portion into your containers and this makes an excellent snack or salad topper.

Spicy Moroccan Salmon

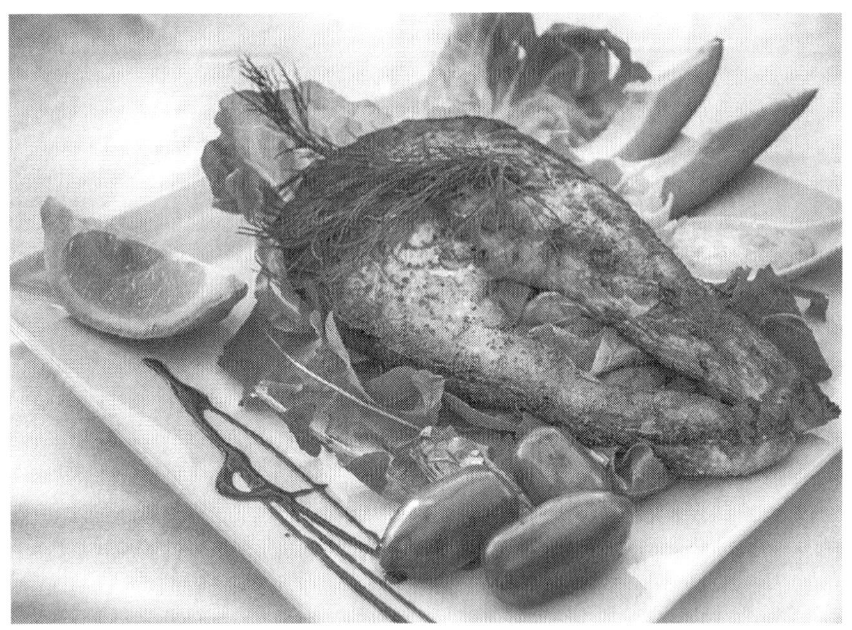

Four Servings
Serving Size: One Salmon Fillet
Carbohydrates: 32g
Proteins: 50g
Fats: 14g

Ingredients:

- Salt (.50 t.)
- Pepper (.50 t.)
- Cilantro (1 T.)
- Salmon Fillets (4)

Sauce:

- Smoked Paprika (1 t.)
- Garlic (3)
- Honey (1 T.)

- Ginger (1.50 t.)
- Lemon Juice (1 T.)
- Olive Oil (1 T.)
- Harissa (3 T.)

Directions:

1. Start off by heating your oven to 400 degrees.
2. Take heavy duty tin foil and lay them out onto a baking sheet.
3. Carefully season the salmon with the salt and pepper and place them skin side down into the tin foil.
4. In a small bowl, mix together all of the sauce ingredients from the list above. Be sure that they are well blended and then spoon them over the fillets of salmon.
5. Fold the tin foil over the fish and bake in the oven for twenty minutes. This should be enough time to cook the salmon through so it is nice and flakey.
6. For some extra flavor, add some chopped cilantro when you portion into your containers.

Chapter Six: Vegetable Recipes

Garlic Roasted Cauliflower

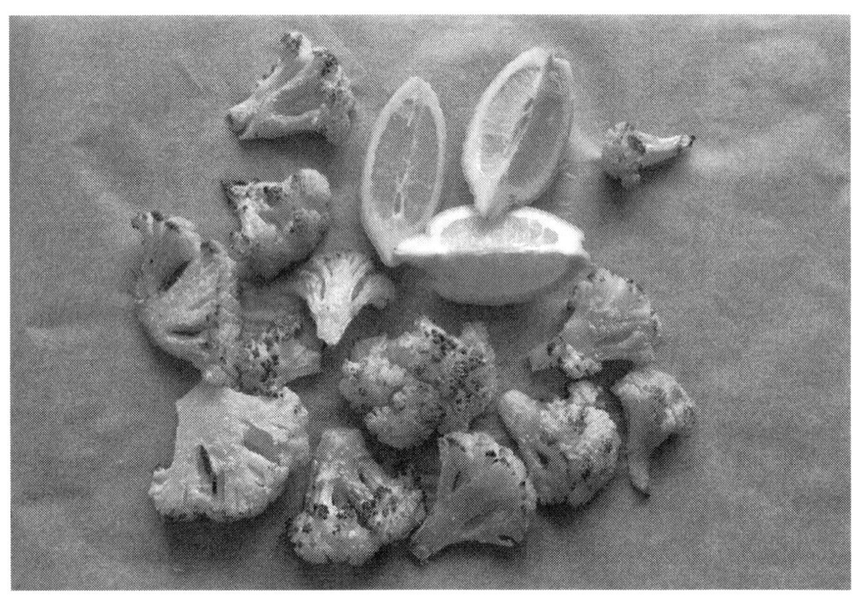

Six Servings
Serving Size: .50 C.
Carbohydrates: 9g
Proteins: 5g
Fats: 9g

Ingredients:

- Parsley (1 T.)
- Salt (.50 t.)
- Pepper (.50 t.)
- Parmesan Cheese (.33 C.)
- Cauliflower (1)
- Olive Oil (3 T.)
- Garlic (2 T.)

Directions:

1. Start out by heating your oven to 450 degrees.

2. While this warms up, take a large baking dish and place your cauliflower. Sprinkle the garlic and olive oil over the top.
3. Finally, season with salt and pepper to taste.
4. Pop the dish into the oven and cook for a total of twenty-five minutes. Halfway through, remove the dish and sprinkle the parmesan cheese on and then broil for five minutes. This will turn the cauliflower a nice golden brown color.
5. Portion out the cauliflower and serve with a favorite protein.

Parmesan Asparagus

Five Servings
Serving Size: .50 C.
Carbohydrates: 5g
Proteins: 8g
Fats:18g

Ingredients:

- Salt (.50 t.)
- Pepper (.50 t.)
- Parmesan Cheese (.75 C.)
- Asparagus (1 Lb.)
- Olive Oil (.25 C.)
- Butter (1 T.)

Directions:

1. Begin by heating a medium skillet over medium heat. Place your tablespoon of butter and olive oil and bring to a sizzle.
2. Once the olive oil and butter are heated, toss in the asparagus and stir for ten minutes.
3. When the asparagus is cooked through, remove any extra oil, sprinkle on the parmesan cheese and salt and pepper to taste.
4. Portion out the asparagus and enjoy with any lunch or dinner for delicious meal prep.

Parsley and Lemon Green Beans
Four Servings
Serving Size: .50 C.
Carbohydrates: 13g
Proteins: 3g
Fats: 9g

Ingredients:

- Lemon (1)
- Salt (.50 t.)
- Pepper (.50 t.)
- Parsley (.25 C.)
- Lemon Zest (1 T.)
- Garlic (3)
- Olive Oil (2 t.)
- Butter (2 T.)
- Green Beans (1 Lb.)
- White Sugar (.10 t.)

Directions:

1. Begin by bringing a pot of water to a boil. Once the water is boiling, toss in a pinch of white sugar and your green beans. Allow these to cook for five minutes or until they are tender.
2. In a large skillet, heat up the olive oil over medium heat. Add in the butter next and allow it to melt before tossing in the garlic and green beans.
3. Season the beans with the parsley, pepper, salt, and lemon zest. Cook this combination for another couple of minutes.
4. Finally, portion out your side dish and enjoy.

Fried Green Tomatoes
Four Servings
Serving Size: .25 C.
Carbohydrates: 57g
Proteins: 13g
Fats: 27g

Ingredients:

- Vegetable Oil (1 Q.)
- Black Pepper (.50 t.)
- Salt (.50 t.)
- Bread Crumbs (.50 C.)
- Cornmeal (.50 C.)
- All-purpose Flour (1 C.)
- Milk (.50 C.)
- Eggs (2)
- Green Tomatoes (4)

Directions:

1. To start, pour the vegetable oil into a large pan and begin to heat it up into a medium heat.
2. While the oil heats, you will want to prepare your tomatoes by slicing them into .50 inch thick pieces. Be sure to throw the ends out as you will have no need for them.
3. In a bowl, mix together the milk and the eggs.
4. Place your flour onto a plate and line up with the bowl that is holding the milk and eggs.
5. On a third plate, mix together your breadcrumbs, cornmeal, pepper, and salt.
6. Now that these are prepared, dip your tomato pieces in the liquid mixture, the flour, and then the breadcrumb mixture. Be sure to coat the tomatoes before tossing them into the vegetable oil.
7. Fry the tomatoes for five minutes on either side or until golden brown.

8. Portion them out and enjoy as a side dish or a nice, healthy snack!

Grilled Herbed Artichokes

Four Servings
Serving Size: .50 C.
Carbohydrates: 19g
Proteins: 6g
Fats: 14g

Ingredients:

- Butter (.25 C.)
- Artichokes (4)
- Lemon (1)
- Salt (1 t.)
- White Wine (.25 C.)
- Olive Oil (1 t.)
- Liquid Smoke Flavor (.50 t.)
- Thyme (.25 t.)
- Basil (.25 t.)
- Italian Seasoning (.50 t.)

Directions:

1. Begin by placing a pot filled with water over medium heat. As the water begins to boil, add in the liquid smoke, white wine, salt, olive oil, basil, thyme, and Italian seasoning.
2. Once this is done, squeeze in the lemon juice and drop the whole thing into the pot.
3. When the water is boiling, toss in the artichoke and cook for thirty minutes.
4. Remove the artichoke from the water, remove any excess water and portion out.

Sweet Glazed Carrots
Eight Servings
Serving Size: 1 C.
Carbohydrates: 18g
Proteins: 2g
Fats: 6g

Ingredients:

- Pepper (.25 t.)
- Salt (.25 t.)
- Brown Sugar (.25 C.)
- Butter (.25 C.)
- Carrots (2 Lbs.)

Directions:

1. To start, pour water into a large saucepan and bring it to a boil. Once the water is boiling, add in the carrots and reduce the heat to simmer the carrots for ten minutes. When the carrots are nice and soft, drain the water and place them into a bowl to the side.
2. In the same saucepan, begin to melt the butter. Once it is melted, add in the pepper, salt, and brown sugar. Gently toss the carrots into the sauce and cook them for five more minutes or so.
3. Finally, turn off the heat and allow the carrots to cool. Place a cup to each container, and you have a great snack or side dish for any lunch or dinner.

Lemon and Garlic Roasted Broccoli
Six Servings
Serving Size: .50 C.
Carbohydrates: 7g
Proteins: 3g
Fats: 2g

Ingredients:

- Lemon Juice (.50 t.)
- Garlic (1)
- Black Pepper (.50 t.)
- Salt (1 t.)
- Olive Oil (2 t.)
- Broccoli (2)

Directions:

1. Begin heating your oven to 400 degrees.
2. In a bowl, mix the pepper, salt, garlic, olive oil, and broccoli all together. Be sure that the broccoli is evenly coated to assure the best flavor.
3. Place the broccoli onto a baking sheet and cook for twenty minutes or until the vegetable becomes soft and tender.
4. Finally, squeeze lemon liberally over the broccoli, portion, and enjoy.

Simple Roasted Asparagus

Four Servings

Serving Size: .50 C.

Carbohydrates: 6g

Proteins: 4g

Fats: 11g

Ingredients:

- Lemon Juice (1 T.)
- Black Pepper (.50 t.)
- Salt (1 T.)
- Garlic (1)
- Olive Oil (3 T.)
- Asparagus (1 Bunch)

Directions:

1. You can start out by heating your oven to 425 degrees.
2. While this warms up, place your asparagus in a bowl and coat it with olive oil. Once it is well covered, toss in the salt, pepper, and lemon juice and be sure to season it well.
3. Finally, place the asparagus onto a baking sheet and pop into the oven for fifteen minutes.
4. Remove from the oven, portion out into your containers, and enjoy your healthy side.

Roasted Butternut Squash
Four Servings
Serving Size: 1 C.
Carbohydrates: 31g
Proteins: 3g
Fats: 7g

Ingredients:

- Salt (.50 t.)
- Pepper (.50 t.)
- Garlic (2)
- Olive Oil (2 T.)
- Butternut Squash (1)

Directions:

1. Start off this recipe by heating your oven to 400 degrees.
2. Next, prepare your butternut squash by cutting it into cubes and tossing in olive oil and garlic. You can also season with salt and pepper if you desire.
3. Finally, arrange the squash onto a baking sheet and cook for thirty minutes or so.
4. Remove the squash from the oven, cool, and portion out into your containers.

Cilantro and Lime Cauliflower Rice

Four Servings
Serving Size: .50 C.
Carbohydrates: 10g
Proteins: 4g
Fats: 6g

Ingredients:

- Butter (2 T.)
- Cilantro (.50 C.)
- Lime (1)
- Water (1 T.)
- Cauliflower (1)

Directions:

1. To start off, you will want to grate the cauliflower. If you have a food processor, stick it in there and pulse until the cauliflower begins to resemble rice.
2. Once it is created, place it in the microwave for seven minutes or so. This should be enough time to make the cauliflower become soft and tender.
3. Finally, remove the rice from the microwave. When it has cooled, toss in the lime juice, lime zest, butter, and cilantro. Mix everything together well and then portion into your containers. This is an excellent carb replacement if you are trying to lose weight.

Chapter Seven: Dessert Recipes

Avocado Chocolate Pudding

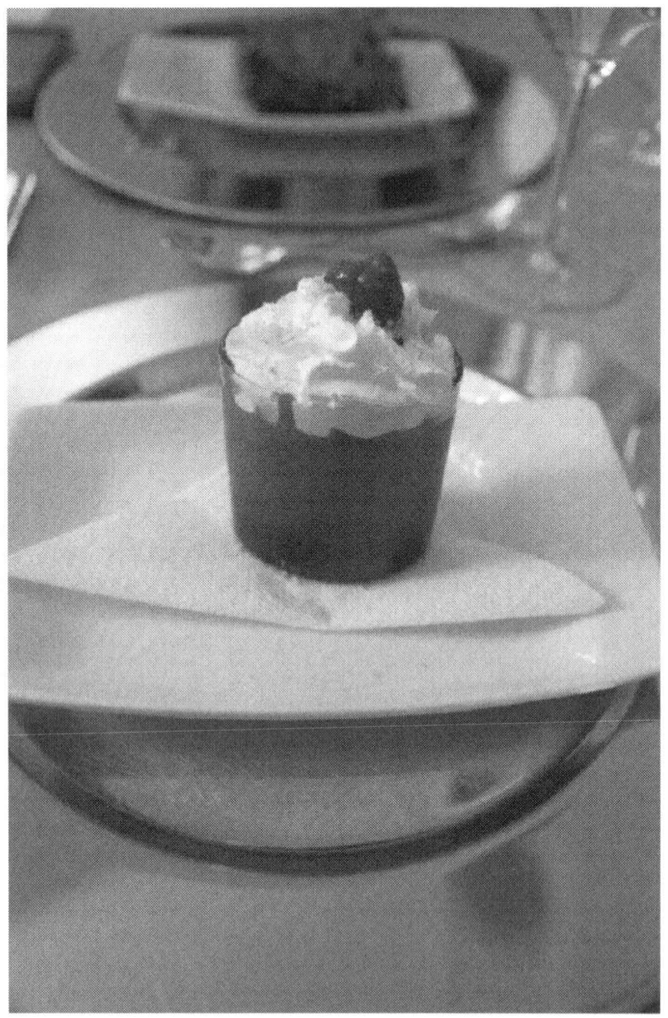

Six Servings
Serving Size: .50 C.
Carbohydrates: 21g
Proteins: 3g
Fats: 10g

Ingredients:

- Salt (.50 t.)

- Vanilla Extract (2 t.)
- Vanilla Almond Milk (.50 C.)
- Greek Yogurt (2 T.)
- Honey (.25 C.)
- Unsweetened Cocoa Powder (.50 C.)
- Avocados (2)

Directions:

1. Simply take all of the ingredients from above and place it into a blender. Pulse the ingredients until they become a creamy, smooth consistency.
2. For some extra flavor, top with your favorite whipped cream. Portion and you have a quick, healthy dessert!

Lemon and Blueberry Bread Pudding
Four Servings
Serving Size: 1 C.
Carbohydrates: 44g
Proteins: 9g
Fats: 5g

Ingredients:

- Blueberries (1 Pint)
- Lemon (1)
- Salt (.25 t.)
- Vanilla Extract (.50 t.)
- Brown Sugar (1 T.)
- Honey (1 T.)
- Eggs (2)
- Unsweetened Applesauce (.50 C.)
- Almond Milk (1.50 C.)
- Whole Wheat Bread (5 C.)

Directions:

1. Begin by heating your oven to 350 degrees.
2. While this warms up, take a small bowl to combine the lemon zest, salt, vanilla extract, brown sugar, honey, eggs, applesauce, and milk. Gently whisk everything together until it is well combined.
3. Next, chop up the bread into two inch cubes. Once this is done, fold the bread and blueberries into the egg mixture.
4. Place all of these ingredients into a bowl and allow to soak in the fridge for an hour or so.
5. Pop the baking dish into the oven for fifty minutes to an hour and cook until it comes out a golden brown color.
6. Portion out the dessert and microwave when you want a healthy dessert.

Pumpkin Spice Mug Cake
One Serving
Serving Size: One Mug Cake
Carbohydrates: 35g
Proteins: 5g
Fats: 1g

Ingredients:

- Vanilla Extract (.25 t.)
- Unsweetened Apple Sauce (1.50 t.)
- Almond Milk (2 T.)
- Pumpkin Puree (2 t.)
- Maple Syrup (1 T.)
- Nutmeg (.10 t.)
- Pumpkin Pie Spice (.25 t.)
- Cinnamon (.25 t.)
- Baking Powder (.50 t.)
- Whole Wheat Flour (4 T.)

Directions:

1. In your favorite mug, first, you will want to mix together all of the dry ingredients from the list above.
2. Once this is done, one by one stir in your wet ingredients. Stir everything together to assure there are no clumps in your cake.
3. Pop the mug into the microwave for one minute.
4. Allow the cake to cool before you enjoy!

Sweet Apple Oatmeal Cider Crisp
Eight Servings
Serving Size: .75 C.
Carbohydrates: 43g
Proteins: 4g
Fats: 10g

Ingredients:

- Cinnamon Sticks (2)
- Maple Syrup (.33 C.)
- Apple Cider (2 C.)
- Apples (6)

Topping:

- Salt (.25 t.)
- Allspice (.25 t.)
- Cinnamon (1 t.)
- Vanilla Extract (1 t.)
- Apple Cider Mix (.25 C.)
- Almond Flour (.50 C and 2 T.)
- Pecans (.50 C.)
- Rolled Oats (1 C.)

Directions:

1. Begin by heating your oven to 375 degrees.
2. While this heats up, begin to prepare your apples by peeling them and slicing them. Once this is done, toss them in a large bowl and set it to the side.
3. Next, take a saucepan and heat it over a high heat. Once it is warm, add in your cinnamon sticks, maple syrup, and apple cider and bring to a boil. When it begins to boil, turn down the heat and simmer this mix for twenty minutes or so.
4. After the time has passed, remove the sticks and pour the warm mixture over the apples. You will want to save .25 C. of this liquid for later use.

5. Once this step has been done, take another bowl and combine the following: salt, allspice, cinnamon, vanilla, apple cider mix, almond flour, pecans, and rolled oats. Be sure to combine everything together well.
6. Next, toss the soaked apples into a baking dish and cover with the crumbled top.
7. Now, it is time to place the baking dish into the oven for thirty minutes.
8. In the end, the recipe will be golden brown. Remove from the oven, allow to cool, and then portion for a healthy dessert option.

Peanut Butter and Apple Cookies

Eighteen Servings
Serving Size: One Cookie
Carbohydrates: 10g
Proteins: 3g
Fats: 6g

Ingredients:

- White Chocolate Chips (.25 C.)
- Apple Pie Spice (.25 t.)
- Ground Flax Seed (2 T.)
- Peanuts (2 T.)
- Dried Apples (.33 C.)
- Rolled Oats (1 C.)
- Rice Cereal (1 C.)
- Vanilla Extract (.50 t.)
- Honey (2 T.)
- Peanut Butter (.33 C.)
- Coconut Oil (4 T.)

Directions:

1. To start out, begin to melt the vanilla, honey, peanut butter, and coconut oil in a saucepan over low heat. Continue to melt this mixture until the ingredients are well blended and smooth.
2. Remove the pan from the heat and stir in all other ingredients minus the white chocolate chips.
3. Now, take the mixture and create small balls. Place these onto a baking sheet and pop them into the fridge for twenty minutes.
4. For some extra flavor, melt the white chocolate chips and drizzle over the top.
5. Portion out the cookies and save for a sweet treat.

Simple Chocolate Chip Cookies
Fifteen Servings
Serving Size: Two Cookies
Carbohydrates: 17g
Proteins: 4g
Fats: 10g

Ingredients:

- Dark Chocolate Chips (.50 C.)
- Vanilla Extract (1 t.)
- Honey (.25 C.)
- Coconut Oil (5 T.)
- Eggs (2)
- Salt (.25 t.)
- Baking Soda (1 t.)
- Almond Flour (.50 C.)
- Whole Wheat Flour (1.50 C.)

Directions:

1. Start off by heating your oven to 350 degrees.
2. While this warms up, line a cookie sheet with parchment paper, so it is ready.
3. Now, take a small bowl and mix together the baking soda, almond flour, whole wheat flour, and set it to the side.
4. In a mixer, blend together the vanilla, honey, coconut oil, and eggs. As this blends, slowly add in the flour mixture until everything is well combined.
5. When you are ready, fold in the dark chocolate chips and carefully spoon a tablespoon of this mixture onto the cooking sheet. There should be about thirty balls at the end.
6. Pop the cookie sheet into the oven for ten minutes or until they are a nice golden color.
7. Remove the cookies from the oven, cool, and portion out!

Quinoa and Peanut Butter No Bake Balls
Twelve Servings
Serving Size: One Ball
Carbohydrates: 17g
Proteins: 5g
Fats: 6g

Ingredients:

- Salt (.10 t.)
- Cinnamon (.50 t.)
- Vanilla Extract (1 t.)
- Maple Syrup (.25 C.)
- Peanut Butter (.33 C.)
- Sunflower Seeds (.25 C.)
- Raisins (.33 C.)
- Coconut, Shredded (3 T.)
- Rolled Oats (1 C.)
- Cooked Quinoa (1 C.)

Directions:

1. Start off by mixing all of the ingredients together in a bowl. If you have a blender, this will make it even easier.
2. Once the dough is formed, roll the mix into balls and place them on a pan.
3. Pop the pan into the fridge and allow the balls to cool for a couple of hours.
4. These balls are great for a quick snack during the day or a sweet treat when you need one.

Thin Funfetti Cookies
Thirty Servings
Serving Size: One Cookie
Carbohydrates: 15g
Proteins: 1g
Fats: 2g

Ingredients:

- Eggs (2)
- Vanilla Yogurt (.50 C.)
- Funfetti Cake Mix (1 Box)

Directions:

1. Start off by heating your oven to 375 degrees.
2. While this warms up, mix together the cake mix with the eggs and the fat-free yogurt. Mix everything together until there are no longer clumps.
3. Next, take out a cookie sheet and cover with tin foil. Carefully spoon out the mix onto the cookie sheet and pop into the oven for twelve minutes or so.
4. Remove cookies when they turn brown on the bottoms, portion, and enjoy a small treat.

Skinny Watermelon Icey Pops
Twelve Servings
Serving Size: One Pop
Carbohydrates: 17g
Proteins: 1g
Fats: 2g

Ingredients:

- Lime Sherbet (1 Pint)
- Mini Chocolate Chips (.25 C.)
- Sugar (.50 C.)
- Watermelon Pulp-Seeded (5 C.)

Directions:

1. Begin by placing the watermelon and sugar into a blender and pulsing until it becomes smooth. Next, strain this mixture into a bowl and pop into the freezer until the mix becomes slushy. This should take around three hours.
2. Once you have a slush, fold in the chocolate chips and pour into disposable cups. When this step is done, place the cups into your freezer for two hours or so. After two hours, the cups should be solid but not frozen.
3. Now, spread the lime sherbet over the top and insert the Popsicle sticks.
4. For best results, leave the pops in overnight to allow them to freeze completely.

Raspberry and Chocolate Grain-Free Mini Cakes

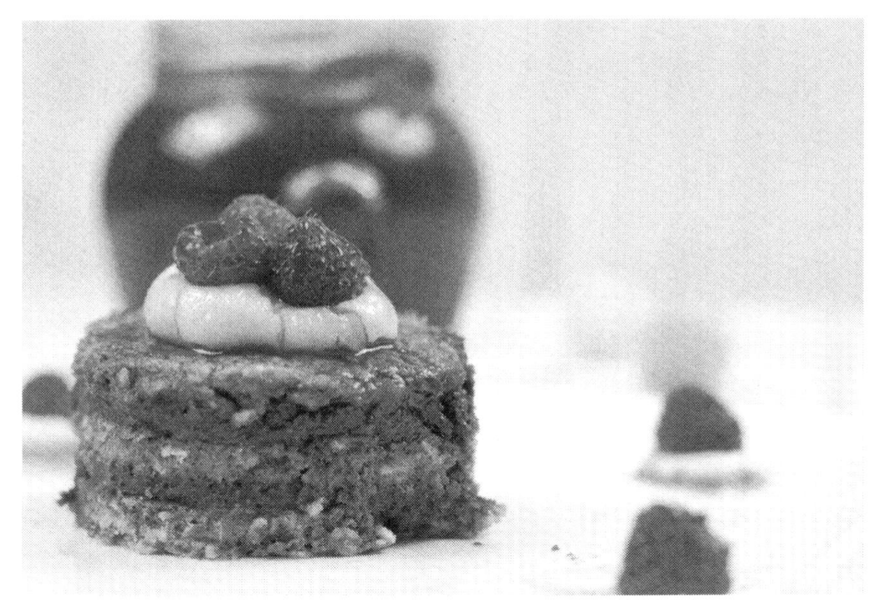

Twelve Servings
Serving Size: One Cake
Carbohydrates: 18g
Proteins: 6g
Fats: 15g

Ingredients:

- Raspberry Preserves (4 T.)
- Maple Syrup (.50 C.)
- Coconut Oil (.25 C.)
- Almond Milk (.50 C.)
- Eggs (3)
- Salt (.25 t.)
- Baking Powder (1.50 t.)
- Cocoa Powder (.75 C.)
- Coconut Flour (2 T.)
- Almond Flour (1.75 C.)
- Fresh Raspberries (1 C.)

Directions:

1. Start off by heating your oven to 350 degrees.
2. While this warms, mix together the coconut flour, almond flour, salt, baking powder, and cocoa powder.
3. In a different bowl, combine the wet ingredients including maple syrup, coconut oil (melted), almond milk, and eggs.
4. Now, combine everything together and fold in the raspberry preserves. Be sure everything is well mixed so that there are no clumps in the mixture.
5. Divide your chocolate batter into greased muffin tins and pop into the heated oven for twenty-five minutes or until baked through.
6. Remove from the oven, cool, and portion for a tasty treat.

Thin Strawberry Cheesecake

Eight Servings
Serving Size: One Slice
Carbohydrates: 29g
Proteins: 4g
Fats: 9g

Ingredients:

- Fresh Strawberries (14)
- Vanilla Extract (2 T.)
- Stevia (6 Packets)
- Reduced-fat Graham Cracker Crust (1)
- Fat-free Cream Cheese (1 Package)
- Cool Whip (8 oz.)

Directions:

1. Start off this recipe by taking a large bowl and mixing together your stevia, vanilla extract, and the cream cheese. You will want to mix these all together until it becomes fluffy. If you want, try to add in some whipped cream to make it even smoother.
2. Next, you will want to spoon this mixture into your pie crust. We suggest using a graham cracker crust, but you can use whatever you like best.
3. Once in place, toss the pie into the fridge for a few hours or until it becomes firm.
4. While the pie firms in the fridge, prep your strawberries by cutting the tops off and cutting them long ways into halves.
5. Finally, remove the pie from the fridge and gently place the strawberry pieces.
6. Slice up the pie, and you have a healthy and delicious dessert for when you need it!

Conclusion

I hope at this point in the book, you are feeling a bit more confident about meal prepping. Remember that this isn't something you have to DIVE into. It is perfectly okay to plan on one meal for the week. This one meal is better than no meals at all. Slowly, you will become surer of your skills and be able to advance to prepping multiple meals in a week. Whether you are doing this for yourself, or your whole family, remember all of the incredible benefits that come with meal prepping!

If you ever feel lost, be sure to refer back to the very first chapter of this book. It will cover all of the basics including tips and tricks, pros and cons, and the basic schedule to follow. If you take anything away, remember to choose a day and take the time. It may seem like you are spending a lot of time cooking but remember that you will be saving that cooking and prepping time through your whole week. Now, you can focus on what you will spend all of this extra time doing! Perhaps it will be taking that exercise class you've been thinking about or some quality family time. Either way, meal prepping can shed new light on a healthier lifestyle.

Hopefully, you have found at least one recipe within these chapters you are excited to try. I tried my very best to include a wide variety of meals for you to prep. Whether you are vegan, vegetarian, or eat everything, there is a recipe out there for you. As I said before, try to start simple. Perhaps grab a breakfast recipe like the overnight oats blueberry muffin style or a simple detox ginger and peach smoothie. The best part is that it is up to you! There is so much flexibility with meal prep, all it takes is a little time and dedication.

If you enjoyed what you learned in this book, it would be appreciated if you would leave a five-star review. The goal is to help as many people out there as possible. I understand that meal prepping can be overwhelming, which is why I have created this book in the first place. Now, I wish you the best of luck on your health journey and remember to enjoy it along the way.

15403659R00062

Printed in Great Britain
by Amazon